Project Management of Clinical Trials

Project Management of Clinical Trials

Richard Chamberlain

Copyright © 2019 by Richard Chamberlain.

Library of Congress Control Number:		2019908132
ISBN:	Hardcover	978-1-7960-4157-6
	Softcover	978-1-7960-4158-3
	eBook	978-1-7960-4159-0

All rights reserved. No part of this book may be reproduced or transmitted in any form or by any means, electronic or mechanical, including photocopying, recording, or by any information storage and retrieval system, without permission in writing from the copyright owner.

The information, ideas, and suggestions in this book are not intended as a substitute for professional medical advice. Before following any suggestions contained in this book, you should consult your personal physician. Neither the author nor the publisher shall be liable or responsible for any loss or damage allegedly arising as a consequence of your use or application of any information or suggestions in this book.

Any people depicted in stock imagery provided by Getty Images are models, and such images are being used for illustrative purposes only. Certain stock imagery © Getty Images.

Print information available on the last page.

Rev. date: 09/24/2019

To order additional copies of this book, contact:
Xlibris
1-888-795-4274
www.Xlibris.com
Orders@Xlibris.com

Dedicated to friends I work with
To contribute to Positive HealthCare

Contents

1. **Introduction** 1
2. **What is Project Management?** 5
   - 2.1 State of the industry 5
   - 2.2 Initiating projects 9
   - 2.3 Planning projects 10
   - 2.4 Resources 11
   - 2.5 Dates 11
3. **What is a Clinical Trial?** 15
   - 3.1 Organization 15
   - 3.2 Personnel 17
   - 3.3 Documentation 18
4. **Some Other Requirements** 23
   - 4.1 Key Words 24
   - 4.2 Quality Assurance and Quality Control 25
   - 4.3 Products 27
   - 4.4 Procedures 28
   - 4.5 Regulations 29
   - 4.6 Compliance 31
   - 4.7 Documentation 31
   - 4.8 Risk Management 33
   - 4.9 Risk-Based Monitoring 38
5. **The management of Clinical Trials** 41
   - 5.1 What are Trials? 41
   - 5.2 Produce the Plan 43
   - 5.3 What is in Scheduling a Visit? 48

6. **Planning a Trial** 55
   6.1 Estimation of Study Dates, Resources, and Costs 58

7. **Estimating Costs and Resources using Excel** 73
   7.1 Use Excel or MS Project 73
   7.2 An Example with Excel 74
   7.3 "Default Values" 74
   7.4 Study Effort 75
   7.5 Execute and Control the Clinical Plans 75
   7.6 Start-up Resources 76
   7.7 Gantt Chart 77
   7.8 Execute and Control the Clinical Plans Monthly
       Projections 77

8. **The Excel Worksheets** 81

9. **Managing a Trial** 89
   9.1 Study Start-up 93
   9.2 Study Execution 94
   9.3 Study Close-out 95
   9.4 Making Adjustments to the Plan 96
   9.5 Making Changes to the Spreadsheets 97
   9.6 Adding a new "Standard" Trial 97
   9.7 Deleting a Standard Trial 97
   9.8 Adding a new Resource 98
   9.9 Adding a New Study 98

10. **Valid Processes** 101
    10.1 Process Validation 102
    10.2 Process Management and Project Management 104

11. **Development of SOPs** 107
    11.1 Identifying the SOP 107
    11.2 History of Revisions 108
    11.3 SOP Sections 109
    11.4 Length and Detail 111
    11.5 Contents 112
    11.6 Reviews 112
    11.7 SOP on SOPs 112

12. Sample SOPs 113

13. If All Else Fails 123

Appendix A – Quality Management 125
    A Processes 128
    B Personnel 132
    C Projects 133

Acknowledgements

I want to thank my Daughters and their families.

I received encouragement from them and numerous other people as I prepared this. I wish to thank them all.

The "sayings" at the beginning of each chapter are from the website;

http://www.devrand.com/

1. Introduction

Conducting a clinical trial can be a large complicated project that is fraught with several complicated, difficult questions. A clinical trial is covered by FDA (and some other) regulations, and it is expected to be sensitive to the Quality of the treatment the patient is receiving.

The conduct of the clinical trial can also involve a variety of different organizations such as Diagnostic laboratories, pharmacies, other laboratories, hospital review boards, and others.

This publication is organized into several sections. The first section is covered by the following four chapters. The chapters cover the following;

Chapter 2 – An introduction to Project Management. What are the various aspects to project management that impact the conduct of a clinical trial? The main resource we use is the book published by the Project Management Institute – Project Management Body of Knowledge (PMBOK). We will look at a couple of other sources too but the main thrust is from PMBOK.

Chapter 3 – An introduction to what is a Clinical Trial. There are different kinds of clinical trials but there are a lot of similarities.

We will go through both the similarities and the differences and describe, in general, how clinical trials are conducted.

Chapter 4 – What are some other requirements that apply to all clinical trials? These are things like Quality Assurance and Quality Control, applicable regulations and compliance to those regulations, the use of Risk Management to determine how some things are done, and Cost and Resource issues.

Chapter 5 – How do we put those three chapters together as we manage clinical trials? We have included the use of an Excel spreadsheet for much of the scheduling, resource and cost management. This spreadsheet is available for your own use. It is not "locked" and can be edited or tailored to your products, your staff, your environment, and so on.

The first four chapters should give you a good start at managing your trials. The next three chapters go into more detail regarding estimating tracking resources, costs, and dates. As was mentioned, starting in chapter 7 an Excel spreadsheet will be used to manage this information. It was also mentioned that something like MS Project could also be used. You should look at what is done here and then decide what would work best for you. Chapter 10 will discuss "managing" trials based on this information.

Chapter 6 – Tracking Study Progress; the development of a report to begin to track the progress of your clinical trials. A report like the one proposed here can form the basis for the more detailed reporting and tracking (management) that follows.

Chapter 7 – Estimating the Study Budget, Resources and Costs – Based on the above report how do we estimate monthly resources and monthly costs for our trials?

Chapter 8 – Estimating Costs and Resources using Excel. MS Project could also be used for this reporting. We chose to use Excel because some of the reporting is easier to do. MS Project tends to do a lot of reporting "Automatically" which may not be the exact information we need in this case.

Chapter 9 – The Excel Spreadsheets – Directions on how to modify the Excel Spreadsheets to match your studies, your personnel, and your practices.

Chapter 10 – Managing a Trial; given the above information what things can you do to manage the trial?

When conducting a clinical trial you should be following a *Process*. The remaining three chapters discuss things like "What is a Valid process?", "How do you develop Procedures to document the Steps used in the process?" These are important because they will be used to determine things like quality, compliance, costs, etc.

Chapter 11 – Valid Processes – Considering topics like Quality and Regulations the definition of *Processes* used to accomplish the tasks is very important. The notion of *Valid* processes becomes very important.

Chapter 12 – Sample SOPs

Chapter 13 – Development of SOPs – When working in a regulated environment documented, approved, procedures become very important.

Appendix A – Quality Management – In some circles the International Standards Organization (ISO) 9000 Standard contains a lot of related, useful practices.

2. What is Project Management?

2.1 State of the industry

When looking at project management there are several resources that apply to managing projects. Consider the following.

- Project Management Institute (PMI) – Body of Knowledge (PMBOK)
- Institute for Electronic and Electrical Engineers (IEEE) – Software Engineering Standards
- Carnegie Melon Institute – Computer Maturity Model
- Agile – Use a version that produces Documentation – e.g. *Agile User Story*
- Others

Project Management Institute publication Body Of Knowledge (PMBOK) says that a project can create;

- A product that can be either a complement of another item an enhancement of an item or an end item in itself;
- A service or a capability to perform a service (e.g. a business function that supports production or distribution);
- An improvement in the existing product or service lines (e.g. a six sigma project undertaken to reduce defects);

- A result, such as an outcome or document (e.g. a research project that develops knowledge that can be used to determine whether a trend exists or a new process will benefit society).

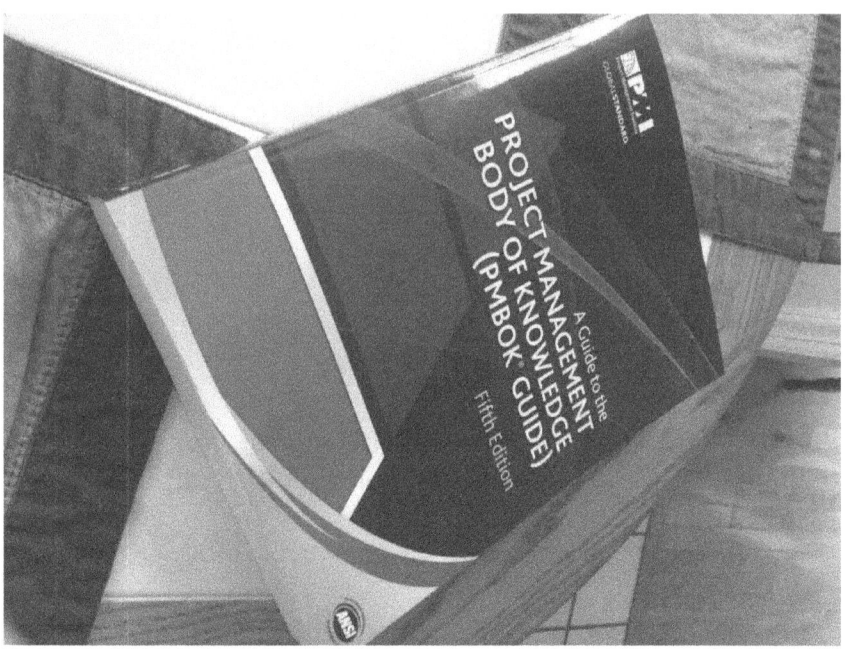

The PMI recommends preparation of a Project Life Cycle that lists the phases that you go through to complete the project.

The PMI shows a sample life cycle made up of the following phases.

- Requirements
- Feasibility
- Planning
- Design
- Construct
- Test
- Turnover

The IEEE Software Engineering Standards has the following Systems Development Life Cycle (SDLC) that they use as an example in their standards. Both the PMI and IEEE discussions on how to prepare a Project Life Cycle.

- Plan
- User Requirements Specifications (URS)
- System Design Specifications (SDS)
- Construction
- Release
- Installation and Acceptance
- System Use
- Archival

If we consider Clinical Research, one way to look at what has to be done might be to consider the development of a New Drug Application (NDA) as the project.

There is extensive documentation available from the FDA on how to do this. The regulations have extensive information and the FDA has extensive Guidance Documents that go further.

You would develop a detailed plan for the preparation of the NDA. In many cases you would even have the plan approved by the FDA before or as you are starting.

This plan would contain a detailed list of the products that would be contained in the NDA. One of these lists would be the list of Clinical Trials that would be conducted.

- A product that can be either a complement of another item an enhancement of an item or an end item in itself;

The clinical trials would be Complements to the NDA and each would be treated as a project.

Project Management Life Cycle (PMBOK)

PMBOK	Clinical Trial
Starting the Project	Plan for the NDA
Organizing and Preparing	Study Start
Carrying out the work	Study Execution
Closing the Project	Study Close-out

The life cycle we recommend using for a clinical trials would be

- Study Planning – Include requirements to satisfy required regulations.

- Study Start – Identify the sites and patients for each site, train all personnel involved in the trial. Set up the medication procedures and laboratory procedures including and diagnostic procedures for the study. This Phase would end when the first patient has their first visit.

- Study Execution – This phase would start when the first patient has their first visit and would end when the last patient has their last visit. During this phase the patients are dosed as required by the protocol and all medical information is collected and processed also as described in the protocol.

- Study Close-out – This Phase will start after the last patient has their last visit. It would finish when the required summaries of results are completed. This includes any required approvals.

2.2 *Initiating projects*

The PMBOK states

Managing a project typically includes, but is not limited to;

- Identifying requirements;
- Addressing the various needs, concerns, and expectations of the stakeholders in planning and executing the project;
- Setting up, maintaining, and carrying out communications among stakeholders that are active, effective, and collaborative in nature;
- Managing stakeholders towards meeting project requirements and creating project deliverables;
- Balancing the competing project constraints, which include, but are not limited to;
    - Scope,
    - Quality,
    - Schedule,
    - Budget,
    - Resources, and
    - Risks

Some potential opportunities;

- Funding, Resources

    Take a realistic look at amount of money budget for the project as well as the number of people available to work on the project.

- Often Starting Project Before you have Requirements

    Do you know everything that will be needed for the project?

- Contingencies – What could go wrong and what if it does?

As you plan the project ask if there are some things that are not known very well. Do a Risk Management of these areas.

- The "Double Rule"

    If the project is new to your staff or if there seem to be some unknowns, you might consider what I call the "Double Rule", that is, double all of the costs and times. I am often amazed at how accurate that is.

- Sit Down Around the Table

    Communication is very important for most projects. Periodically have at least the key individuals involved in the project sit down around the table and go through the project status.

2.3 Planning projects

- Collect as much Information as Possible

    Try to review as much information as is available.

- How Much New Technology – mHealth

    New technology is currently a very concerning issue for many projects. Information is being collected "automatically". Is it the correct information? Consider looking at mHealth or m-Health.

- Adaptive Clinical Trials

    The FDA now allows studies to change (or adapt) during the execution of the study. This can introduce some planning issues. It may be difficult to forecast when the change might occur and what the ramification of those changes might be.

- What Regulations – Foreign?.

  Are there any relevant regulations particularly any foreign regulations? Are there any other "rules" that are required to be followed?

2.4 Resources

- What Resources

  What resources are required to perform the project? It is important to look at all resources. Not only the people but also equipment, supplies, buildings, and others.

- What Responsibilities

  When looking at the personnel resources, is it clear what the responsibilities of each person is? Is it documented and is any training required?

- Clear Assignments

  When the people are assigned and the responsibilities are known is it clear which responsibilities are assigned to each person?

2.5 Dates

- Any Slack?

  Start and completion dates are typically very important for most projects. When setting these dates are there any that have some slack where they can be delayed without impacting the project?

- Dependencies

    Are all relationships between the dates known?

Now consider further definition of what a clinical trial is.

-- Notes --

-- Notes --

3. What is a Clinical Trial?

3.1 Organization

The goal of a clinical trial is to demonstrate the Safety and/or Safety and Efficacy of the treatment being tested. Since we are testing this in human subjects, the *Quality* of the conduct of the trial and the information being observed is very important.

Each clinical trial should be viewed as a *project*. To satisfy the above requirements it is important to apply project management principles to implementing these clinical trials.

The definition of a clinical trial from the National Cancer Institute (NCI.com) is:

> Clinical Trial
>
> A type of research study that tests how well new medical approaches work in people. These studies test new methods of screening, prevention, diagnosis, or treatment of a disease. Also called clinical study.

The National Institute of Health (NIH) also has a very thorough and understandable discussion of what is Clinical Research and <u>What</u> is a Clinical Trial.

http://www.nhlbi.nih.gov/studies/clinicaltrials/

This web site is highly recommended if you are new to this.

The conduct of a clinical trial can involve the following organizations;

The Sponsor – This is the organization that is responsible for the study. They have defined what information is to be observed and analyzed. They have documented all of the procedures that will be followed as the trial is conducted. Typically, they are also the group that pays for the study.

Contract Research Organization (CRO) – As the name implies, this is an organization that is being contracted to do some or all of the study. The responsibility for the study will still lie with the sponsor but the CRO will be doing some (or all) of the work.

A note worth mentioning is that although the CRO is being contracted to do some of the work, it has been our experience that they will still need to be "managed" by the sponsor.

The Clinical Site – This is the group that actually sees the subjects, makes and records the observations required for the study. Each site involved in the trial will have a "Principle Investigator" who will be responsible for the conduct of the study at that site. They will be asked to "sign" the information collected for each subject.

Support functions – The Pharmacy might supply the drug. There might be a laboratory or laboratories that analyze samples. There might be other diagnostic laboratories that are used for the study. These organizations are all required to follow certain FDA regulations.

The sponsor will be responsible for preparation of all documentation required for a New Drug Application (NDA) to get approval to use the treatment in the public. The study documentation will be part of this. The requirements for this can be found in the Code of Federal (CFR) Section 21 Part 312. The requirements for Food Devices and other treatments can be found in other Parts of Section 21 of the CFR.

3.2 Personnel

At the Site

Principal Investigator

Each site must have a Principal Investigator who is responsible for the study activities at that site. They should have reviewed the study protocol and resolved any open questions with the sponsor, probably through the study "Monitor".

Nursing Staff
Administrator

Additional Staff
Laboratory
Pharmacy
Other Diagnostic Staff
    X-ray
    MRI

At the Sponsor or CRO

Medical
Clinical Research Associate
Clinical Monitor*
Data Management
Diagnostic Specialties

Drug Supplies
Regulatory
Legal
Project Management
Laboratory
Statistics
IT

*The Clinical Monitor is very important. This person monitors the activities of the study as it is progressing. This person will likely be a Clinical Research Associate who performs the monitoring. The monitor will travel to the sites and review their activities including a records that are kept. The FDA recently published a Guidance Document entitled "Risk-based Monitoring".

3.3 Documentation

A Drug Study Protocol (from 21 CFR Part 312.23)

A protocol is required to contain the following, with the specific elements and detail of the protocol reflecting the above distinctions depending on the phase of study:

(a) A statement of the objectives and purpose of the study.

(b) The name and address and a statement of the qualifications (curriculum vitae or other statement of qualifications) of each investigator, and the name of each subinvestigator (e.g., research fellow, resident) working under the supervision of the investigator; the name and address of the research facilities to be used; and the name and address of each reviewing Institutional Review Board.

(c) The criteria for patient selection and for exclusion of patients and an estimate of the number of patients to be studied.

(d) A description of the design of the study, including the kind of control group to be used, if any, and a description of methods to be used to minimize bias on the part of subjects, investigators, and analysts.

(e) The method for determining the dose(s) to be administered, the planned maximum dosage, and the duration of individual patient exposure to the drug.

(f) A description of the observations and measurements to be made to fulfill the objectives of the study.

(g) A description of clinical procedures, laboratory tests, or other measures to be taken to monitor the effects of the drug in human subjects and to minimize risk.

A Statistical Analysis Plan (SAP)

This plan will go into more detail regarding the study design and the planned analysis.

Statistical Report

A stand-alone report the produces the Results of the Statistical Analysis. The results of this report will typically be used as input to the Clinical Study report.

Data Management Plan (DMP)

This document will contain the details of all data entry procedures. There will be descriptions on any size or range limitations, special characters, and any editing procedures to detect bad or suspect values.

Study Report(s)

Typically there will be one study report that describes all of the study results. This report should match what was presented in the study protocol.

Other Study Records

The project team should consider what records are generated during the trial that might be needed for regulatory or other reasons and make certain those records are accounted for.

– Notes –

4. Some Other Requirements

Given the above introduction to Project Management and the conduct of Clinical Trials there are some key concepts that need to be understood and have to be included in what is done as you manage the clinical trials as projects.

For example, virtually all of the work above is covered by **regulations**. Largely Food and Drug Association (FDA) regulations but there are a few others too.

The notion of **Quality** permeates everything. Experimental medications or other treatments are being administered to human subjects. The safety of the patient is paramount to everything that is done. Therefore, the notions of Quality Assurance and Quality Control are applied to all steps in our projects.

Since we are seeing human patients we want to minimize the **Risk** to the patient. In other words are we managing all of the risks in the treatments the patients are receiving?

There are a few other things too.

4.1 Key Words

Since we are discussing the execution of clinical trials and that is occurring in a "regulated" environment we are going to introduce some topics that are "related" to the conduct of a clinical trial but are a requirement because of these regulations.

- Quality Assurance and Quality Control – Wring down what to do, doing it and then reviewing the results to see if any improvements can be made.

- Procedures – What are the steps that need to be followed?

- Products – What products are produced as the procedures are followed? These can be paper or electronic.

- Documentation – What documentation exists that can form the basis for what is supposed to be done and what was actually done?

- Regulations – What are the regulations that apply to conducting a clinical Trial?

- Compliance – Compliance is the ability to demonstrate that you are satisfying the regulations and other requirements.

- Risk Management – Since we are dealing with experimental treatments administered to human subjects, being able to manage the risks has become important.

- Risk-Based Monitoring – Study progress is supposed to be *monitored* as the study progresses. The FDA published a guidance document describing a monitoring approach based on risks.

Most of these topics have to do with the Quality and Integrity of the study results. This is dealt with by the proper use of things like tools like the Project Management Institute (PMBOK), Institute of Electrical and Electronic Engineers Software Engineering Standards (IEEE), and International Standards Organization (ISO) 9000.

We will start with an introduction to the following concepts before we get into managing a clinical trial.

4.2 *Quality Assurance and Quality Control*

Quality is a very important concept that runs through all of the things we will be doing when we conduct a clinical trial. We will use the ISO 9001 as the basis for our approach.

There is a point regarding Quality that is often over looked. That point is that to really do Quality Management you and almost everyone in the organization has to live and breathe Quality.

Quality has to be a way of life. It has to permeate almost everything and everyone. This is based on actual history by the icons of Quality.

During W. Edwards Deming's time, one of his contemporaries, Walter Shewhart fostered the notion that Quality was P-D-C-A. Where the letters stand for

   Plan – Do – Check – Act

The idea being that you plan what you are going to do. Then you do it according to that plan. Then you *Check* it to see if it is all correct, and then Act based on what you see.

Deming referred to this as a "corruption". He said it should be P-D-S-A. Where you Plan what you are going to do. Then you Do it according to that plan. Then you **Study** it to see if you really are doing things the best way, and then Act based on what you see. Essentially, there is more to it than just checking. You need to really consider everything you are doing to see if there is not a better way.

Throughout his work he tried to implant quality throughout an organization.

There is another reference "*Well Made in America*" which is the story of the recovery of Harley Davidson. Harley Davidson almost went out of business in the 1970's. It was bought by AMF (the bowling people). After a couple of years about a dozen mangers in AMF raised some money, bought Harley Davidson back and took it public. At the same time they decided to improve the quality of the bikes. The quality of the bikes was really bad. They said one year the paint jobs were so bad that as people walked by them in the show room, the air would make the paint flake off and fall on the floor. They also said that 50% of the bikes coming off the assembly line would not start.

They went through a lot of effort and now Harley Davidson motor bikes are arguably some of the highest quality bikes on the market. [I know because I owned one.]

In the book above they said they attributed the success of increasing the quality to three things.

The first was called "EI" or Employee Involvement. They found that they had to involve everyone in the increase of Quality. You cannot assign Quality to a focus group in the corner and everyone else keeps on working.

The second was "JIT" which stands for Just In Time which was in inventory procedure. The problem was that 50% of the materials they were receiving from their suppliers was bad. So what do you do in that situation? They ordered twice as much as they needed and were building huge, worthless inventories. Essentially, they had a lot of bad procedures.

The third thing they attributed the success to was Statistical Quality Control. And the thing they said they did wrong was, they implemented QC last and they should have done it first.

That is, that Quality involves everyone. It has to become a "way of life" for it to be effective. It is not something you can assign to a group in the corner.

4.3 *Products*

The output of the Process will be some products that are required for the business practices (e.g. QA) or the regulations. They might be documentation, that describes some aspect of the product or they might be "Documented Evidence" that something occurred a certain way.

In between the Process and the Products will be two things, Procedures and Projects. The Procedures will be a more detailed description of what the Products are and how to produce them.

It is important that the products produced by the process be periodically reviewed for accuracy. Are they what they are supposed to be?

When the procedures and products produced are reviewed it is important to maintain a "count" or "measure" of how good they are. This forms the basis for determining if the Quality is improving or not. It is important to have a measure of that performance.

These reviews can be very much like what an auditor would do, as a matter of fact some organizations will conduct what they call "Internal Audits" to determine how well the procedures are being followed and are the products what they are supposed to be.

These reviews and measurements will also indicate how well you are "Complying" with relevant regulations.

4.4 *Procedures*

Much of what we do in a regulated industry requires that you have written procedures that you can demonstrate you are following. In other words; are you complying with the Requirements of the Procedures? These are referred to as Standard Operating Procedures (SOP).

Similarly there will, in general, be two types of Procedures;

1. Continuous Procedures
2. Single Result Procedures

The continuous procedures are those that involve a series of steps that are simply executed in a given situation. For example, seeing a patient should be something that involves a series of steps that are known and are executed each time a patient is seen. The procedure will produce a set of Products (results) that will be required to be stored and maintained.

A single Result procedure is one that is intended to produce a product that can be used in the Process, producing a Procedure that is needed for the Process. For example this might be a computer system for something such as reporting serious adverse events. There needs to be procedures that describe how to develop and implement a computer system that will support a Procedure for reporting serious adverse events. This Project will produce Products that are required to support the Process.

The above Project will go on for the life of the system. It will be necessary to maintain the system as changes are required over the life of the system. There will be projects that have a much shorter life. For example, an unexpected event might happen that requires a "Project" to address. This might involve doing something in Excel or SAS to obtain the required answer. Once the result is obtained and "completed" the project would end.

Note: Obviously, there are other terms that could be used and other ways of interpreting those terms. If a different set of terms is more suited to your organization, business practices, or regulations you should feel free to make the necessary modifications.

Keep in mind that there has to be "<u>documentation</u>" that describes the steps defined above and those steps need to leave "<u>evidence</u>" of what actually is done. Without these Compliance is impossible.

4.5 Regulations

Understanding the role of the regulations, their source, and their importance is vital to the way we conduct clinical trials. The Code of Federal Regulations (CFR) Section 21 has all of the Food and Drug Regulations.

If one looks at the history of FDA regulations in the US there are several things to note.

1. The Regulations are Retrospective, not Prospective

    Virtually all of the regulations are in response to some problem. The first regulation was the Biologics Act of 1906. This was because some contaminated diphtheria anti-toxin was accidently distributed to some children, many of whom died. The second set of regulations came in 1938 when a pediatrician used ant-freeze to make liquid forms of sulfa drugs. More regulations came in 1962 with the Kefauver Amendments with the use of Thalidomide for morning sickness which led to serious birth defects. More recent regulations are also because of problems reported in the use of drugs that are approved for sale.

    The implication of this for us is that it usually is not all that informative to look to the regulations for direction on "How to be Compliant". That detail is more a function of your products, your procedures, your staff, your facilities, and more.

2. The Regulations are considered to also be Best Business Practice.

   The FDA will state that the regulations are what you should be doing anyway; that they really do not reflect additional burdens.

3. You Should Accept Ownership of the Regulations

   The best practice for you is to study the regulations and decide what the implications are for you and your business. What do they mean for what you do and how you do it?

   This means getting at least a few people in your organization familiar with the regulations and their "Intent". These people should also follow the regulations because from time to time they change.

4. Guidance Documents

   Along with the Regulations, the FDA publishes Guidance documents that are intended to expand or clarify certain regulations or parts of the regulations. These guidance documents all have a disclaimer at the front that indicates that they are not law and are not required to be followed, but it is a good idea to review them and take advantage of their contents if it applies to you.

The FDA regulations are in the Code of Federal Regulations (CFR) Section 21. Most of the Drug regulations are in Part 300. The initial Parts of the Section 21 are general regulations that apply to Food, Drugs, Devices, and the other areas covered by the FDA.

It is recommended that anyone involved in interpreting these regulations become familiar with the FDA web site www.FDA.Gov. It can be very helpful.

4.6 Compliance

One definition of the word Compliance is the following;

> Compliance is the ability to demonstrate that you are operating according to a set of rules (or regulations).

Notice it includes the phrase "the ability to demonstrate". In other words there has to be *documentation* or some other kind of *product* to show that you are operating according to certain rules or regulations.

These rules typically generate a series of steps derived to make it possible for us to "follow" the rules and produce the desired product. Many of us follow good business practices. The regulatory bodies will argue that the regulations are just good business practice. In any case there is an underlying "process" that has been defined that we try to follow and this process is designed to have us satisfy any business or regulatory "requirements".

When we have a series of steps like these that we follow, the questions can be asked "Are you following the process?" and "Are you producing the desired product?", "Can you show that you are?"

4.7 Documentation

One good way to show you are following the process and producing the desired result is to use Quality Assurance (QA) practices.

The key to each of the three concepts – Compliance, Processes, and Quality Assurance – is *documentation*.

Project Management of Clinical Trials

When I studied for my Ph.D., I was asked by my Major Professor to prove a theorem. My Major Professor was a fairly well known statistician named Oscar Kempthorne. He was having a dispute with a colleague at the time. I could see how, if the theorem was true, then his colleague was wrong. I spent a year trying to prove that theorem, then one day the light went on and I wondered if perhaps the theorem was not true. I had done enough research that I came up with a counter example to show the theorem was not true and I could see a year's worth of research and my Ph.D. going down the drain. Anyway, the research I had been doing also showed me how to rewrite the theorem so it was true and fortunately for me it still showed his colleague was wrong.

So I wrote this all up and set up a meeting with Kempthorne and walked him through it. When I finished he leaned back in his chair, looked out the window and then turned to me and said "You know Dick, the written word is very <u>unreliable</u>." Then he leaned up so he was right in my face and said "but it is the only thing we have". He was telling me to write it up, and a few months later I was finished.

But he was absolutely right. The documentation trail, products, and other trails we leave after our work is "the only thing we have!"

The questions become;

> What documentation do we need?
> How do we generate the documentation?
> How do we assure that the documentation is accurate?
> How do we Store and Retrieve the documentation?
> Is there some documentation that is not necessary or redundant?
> Do we have to generate a new document or can we reference another document?
> And others

As we get into Processes and Quality the answers to these questions will become clearer.

> *A recommendation; fairly early in becoming compliant your group should sit down and compile a list of the Regulations that apply to you as well as business practices that are meant to be implemented.*

We will discuss compliance to regulations (and other things – business practices)

4.8 Risk Management

Risk is an event that has two characteristics; the likelihood or probability that the event will occur and the severity of the event or how bad the reaction to the event will be. In many cases there is a third value and that is the Probability that you will observe the Event when it happens.

The Likelihood and Severity can both be specified as quantitative values or qualitative values. That is, they can have values for example from 1-20, 20- 50, and 50-100, or they might have values such as mild, moderate, and severe.

Given that this is Risk, what is Risk Management?

4.8.1 Risk analysis

"Risk analysis is the process of defining and analyzing the dangers to individuals, businesses and government agencies posed by potential natural and human-caused adverse events. In IT, a risk analysis report can be used to align technology-related objectives with a company's business objectives. A risk analysis report can be either quantitative or qualitative.

In quantitative risk analysis, an attempt is made to numerically determine the probabilities of various adverse events and the likely extent of the losses if a particular event takes place.

Qualitative risk analysis, which is used more often, does not involve numerical probabilities or predictions of loss. Instead, the qualitative method involves defining the various threats, determining the extent of vulnerabilities and devising countermeasures should an attack occur." – TechTarget.com

The first step is to consider what are the risks? In other words, what Events could happen? Then, what is the Likelihood and what is the severity – either numerically or qualitatively.

Develop scales for the likelihood and severity such as the following;

> Severity – 1. Very Severe, 2. Moderately Severe, 3. Somewhat Severe, 4. Mildly Severe

> Likelihood – 1. Very Likely, 2. Somewhat Likely, 3. Slightly Likely, 4 Not Likely

Given this, it is possible to build the following table

		Likelihood			
		1	2	3	4
Severity	1				
	2				
	3				
	4				

Now the goal is to place entries into the table that will indicate what actions to take to mitigate the risk for each level of Severity and Likelihood.

For Example,

	Likelihood			
	1	2	3	4
Severity 1	A	A	B	B
Severity 2	A	B	B	B
Severity 3	B	B	B	C
Severity 4	B	B	C	C

A =
B =
C =

The goal then is to document what to do in each case. For example,

A = Low likelihood and Low severity. In these cases you might do nothing or do periodic manual checks of the products and processes.

C = High Severity and High Likelihood. You might decide that we are going to change our procedures so that his combination is impossible or you might do 100% sampling of the products.

4.8.2 Risk Mitigation

A systematic reduction in the extent of exposure to a risk and/or the likelihood of its occurrence. Also called risk reduction.

		Severity			
		No Impact	Minimal Impact	Some Impact	Large Impact
Likelihood	Not Likely	A	A	B	B
Likelihood	Could Happen	A	B	B	B
Likelihood	Is Likely	A	B	B	C

If you are still in the development or configuration phase it might be good to have something like;

A = Do nothing because it is unlikely to happen
B = Program edit checks such as Range checks or verify patient is already entered
C = Program "pop-down" list of Valid Values, Require second entry or second verification.

If you are in the Support and Maintenance Phase where the system cannot be changed, then the entries might be something like;

> A = Do nothing because it is unlikely to happen
> B = Take extra steps to increase accuracy such as "Double Key Entry"
> C = Do 100% source data verification

If you are looking at another field the tables above might still be usable. For example, consider the field "number of cigarettes smoked". This is typically a Quality of life question and It is virtually impossible to verify.

In this case it might have Risk values of Could Happen but No Impact. If you are not working on a study of smoking habits, the Risk Analysis/Mitigation would say "don't worry about this one."

4.8.3 Risk Management

For our computer systems we will tie the management of risks into the phases of the life cycle. In other words we will look at risks that could occur during development up to and including UAT. Then we will look at risks that could occur during the Support and Maintenance phase – including change control, and then finally risks that could occur during the decommissioning phase.

For each of those three phases a table like the following will be built and populated by the project team.

Project Management of Clinical Trials

Phase of Life Cycle _____

Risk Title	Risk Description	Likelihood or Probability of Occurrence	Severity or Impact of Occurrence

Suppose the system is one for tracking Adverse Events and risks associated with the "Person doing the entry, enters the wrong value." The Risk will depend on which field is being entered and perhaps what the incorrect value is.

So the Risk might be – The Subject/Patient's name is entered incorrectly.

The likelihood could be on a scale of "Not Likely". "Could happen", "Is Likely". The Severity could be "No Impact:, "Minimal Impact", "Some Impact", "Large Impact".

Phase of Life Cycle _____

Risk Title	Risk Description	Likelihood or Probability of Occurrence	Severity or Impact of Occurrence
Name Entry	The Subject/Patient's name is entered incorrectly.	Could Happen	Minimal Impact

The project team should prepare a list of Risks for each system. These should be summarized in the following three tables. (If the tem decides they need more tables, or fewer, the justifications should be documented).

1. Prior to Go-Live
2. Support and Maintenance including Change Control
3. Decommissioning

Phase of Life Cycle _____

Risk Title	Risk Description	Likelihood or Probability of Occurrence	Severity or Impact of Occurrence

4.9 Risk-Based Monitoring

Most sponsors or CROs will have staff who travel from site to site reviewing or monitoring the activities at each site to assure the site is complying with the procedures of the study. The FDA has encourage monitoring that is based on potential risks to the patients or data quality.

The FDA published a guidance document describing Risk-Based Monitoring (RBM).

Guidance for Industry, Oversight of Clinical Investigations - A Risk-Based Approach to Monitoring.

U.S. Department of Health and Human Services - Food and Drug Administration - August 2013

OMB Control No. 0910-0733

– **Notes** –

5. The management of Clinical Trials

5.1 What are Trials?

The clinical trials that are done today are done to specific FDA regulations. The Emphasis of these trials is Safety first, then after the safety is determined then studies showing efficacy can be performed.

The safety has to be demonstrated first in Normal subjects, then in people with the illness.

Clinical trials can be viewed as different but similar projects. There are different types of studies (projects) but structurally they are very similar. We can apply Project Management principles to each of these studies.

Historically there have been four Phases, Phase I through Phase IV, that the studies go through. Today other phases, Phase 0 and Phase V are being introduced.

Given that the emphasis is Safety first, and then Efficacy the Phases are as follows;

- Phase 0

Since this phase is relatively new, it is still under development. It is intended to provide a fast and safe way to determine the impact of new medications or existing medications on different diseases. We will not go into a lot of detail here even though virtually all of the practices described here would apply to these studies.

- Phase I – Safety in "Normal" Subjects

These are typically studies that have only 50 – 100 subjects and are conducted where the subjects can remain continuously for the length of the study. This is done because there is typically a lot of data that is collected for each subject. Sometimes the data is collected for 24 hour periods. Some hospitals have what is called a Phase I (or Phase II) unit for doing these studies.

Because it is often the first time humans have been treated with the drug or device there is an attempt to collect as much data as possible about the responses.

- Phase II – Safety in "Sick" Subjects

These studies are similar to Phase I but the subjects are people with the disease to be treated but the emphasis is still Safety. So there is still a small number of subjects and they are confined to a research unit where they stay for 24 hours a day.

Having said that, typically this will be the first chance there is to see if the drug works in humans.

- Phase III – Safety and Efficacy in "Sick" Subjects

Phase III studies are the large Safety and Efficacy studies where the treatment will be administered the way it is supposed to be if it was on the market and being prescribed or used under "normal" conditions.

These studies could have several hundred subjects.

- Phase IV – Post-Marketing studies

These studies are conducted after the treatment is approved. Most drugs these days are approved after 2000 to 4000 patients have been studied. Given those numbers it is possible that some serious adverse effects were not detected. Because of that and some recent problems with adverse events, most drugs today are given "Conditional" approvals, conditioned on continuous study of the treatment.

In general, the Phase IV studies are also intended to study other positive results that might indicate other uses for the drug.

- Phase V -

Phase V clinical trials refer to comparative effectiveness research and community-based research. Research is done on data collected. All reported uses are evaluated. Patients are not monitored. Its main focus is to determine integration of a new therapy into wide spread clinical practice.

Although these Phases can be very different, they have some characteristics that are the same for all of them. The individual values will obviously be quite different but the basic parameters are all the same.

5.2 Produce the Plan

Parts of a Plan

We will manage the studies by looking at three different characteristics of all trials. These three characteristics are:

1. Dates.
   What dates that things happen are important and need to be monitored?

2. Costs and Resources
   What costs and resources need to be tracked? Where in the trial are the costs or use of resources more or less that should be?

3. Visits
   What goes on during visits is critical to the success of the trial. There is typically detailed activities for the information being collected that must be done according to the protocol and monitored during the trial. Are these activities being done according to the protocol?

- Dates

There are a handful of key dates that are tracked closely during the trial. They often indicate where there might be a problem.

There are typically three steps that a study goes through. These are;

> Study Start – What activities are associated with the study actually starting?

> Study Execution – The activities associated with seeing the patients and administering treatments.

> Study Close-out – When the patients have all been seen and all study information has been collected, what is associated with completing the data collection and preparing the summaries and reports for the study.

The dates associated with these three activities are typically the following;

Study start – This is when you start to work on the study. It is often a somewhat "soft" date and in many cases is not even tracked. It might be tracked if there are some expenses associated with it, for example, if the study is being done by a CRO, then it might make sense to track start dates.

Study Start Completion and Study Execution Start – This is the date of the first visit by the first patient. It is not unusual to see this referred to as the "Study Execution Start". At the site where the study is starting all necessary documentation must be completed, training must be completed, the arrangements with Labs must be completed, and other preparations for the study must completed and "Signed".

The finish of study start and the beginning of Study Execution are the same date. It is the date that the first patient has the first visit. It is assumed that everything necessary to start the study is complete so the Study Start is finished and the sites are ready to start seeing the patients and collecting the data – Study Execution.

Study Execution Close – The date of the last patient visit. Except for answering some questions, presumably this will be the end of study efforts at the sites.

Study Close out start date will be the same as the Study Execution Close.

The Study Close out will probably have several tasks associated with it that can have dates that are tracked.

During the study close out there will likely be

> Database Lock – All of the study data has been edited, cleaned, and signed off.
>
> Statistical Summary Report – The Statistical report is complete.
>
> Clinical Summary Report – The study results are published.

These activities will also have start and completion dates.

Note; It is not unusual to try and include the results of the Statistical Analyses directly in the Clinical Summary to try and speed things up. If that is done there will be no Statistical Summary Report date.

It might also be useful to do the Statistical Analyses on a preliminary version of the database so that when the final version of the database is complete it may only be a matters of hours to have the Statistical Analyses all complete.

If you are "managing" clinical trials these are the kinds of shortcuts you should look for.

The Study Close out usually completes when the Clinical Summary is complete.

Database Lock – This date may be displayed instead of Study Close. It is the date after which the analysis and reporting can begin and is often more important that the actual end of seeing patients.

Clinical Summary – This will typically be the end of the study efforts.

Study Identification

It will first of all be necessary to identify each study. If you are studying multiple drugs and these drugs all have a list of studies and the studies have multiple sites it will be necessary to develop a naming scheme to identify the drug, the study, and the site.

By the time studies are being defined the drug will have a unique identifier. It is likely that there has been some communication with the FDA or other regulatory or legal group and it is always smart to have a unique identifier for that effort.

Similarly, each study should have a unique identifier. We will just use "STnnnn" for the examples that follow but the ID would likely have an abbreviation for the drug, Phase of study or type of study.

Key Information

Now you should be ready to see specific study information on some or all of the studies in question.

This information might be

The dates and enrollment data could be displayed in reports such as the following.

Key Study Dates (as of mm/dd/yyyy)

Study	Study Start	Study Close	Database Lock	Clinical Summary
Drug 001				
ST001				
ST002				
Drug 002				
ST003				

A report like this might form the basis of starting some clinical Research. It might also be very informative to display progress on the studies before they terminate.

After enrollment has started and to track how well things are starting, a report like the following would be helpful.

Key Study Enrollment – Sites/Patients (as of mm/dd/yyyy)

Study	Sites/ Patients	Planned	Planned Study Start	Planned Clinical Summary
Drug 001				
ST001	2/22	5/120		
ST002	4/34	5/120		
Drug 002				
ST003	1/25	1/200		

Reports such as these can form the basis for tracking studies to look for potential problems. Obviously other columns can be added to track additional information. When focusing on dates the study completion might be the first date one looks for. The other dates can be equally important.

The effort required to sign up sites and the effort required to sign up patients will obviously impact dates.

5.3 *What is in Scheduling a Visit?*

It will be necessary to sign up Sites and then they will have to schedule signing up of subjects. This produces two questions;

1. How long will it take to sign up the sites?
2. How long will it then take to sign up the necessary number of subjects?

These two figures along with the length of the dosing regimen will be critical to determining the over-all length of the study.

These two answers will also determine some very important dates in the schedule. The date the first patient is enrolled in the study will be the start date of the Study Execution Phase. The date that the last patient visit occurs will be the finish date for the Study Execution Phase and will be the Start date for the Study Close out Phase.

What is a Visit?

What activities occur during a visit? This is the first activity in producing our plan. What Tasks are performed by whom and how long will it take?

A visit will have a series of steps that each patient must perform. These steps are usually managed by a physician for nurse.

Each of these steps must be documented and then the physician or nurse must be trained. The training must be documented.

This part of the visit is like preparation and use of Standard Operating Procedures (SOP). Chapters 11 and 12 discuss the development of SOPs and include some examples.

During the visit the patient might be examined and observations made that are entered into the study database. It is likely that other information will also be collected and recorded. It is vital that his information be "handled" in accordance with the study protocol. It is not good to get partway through the study and then discover that some of the information was not observed or recorded accurately.

When managing a clinical trial it vital to monitor what is going on during the visits. Are there study monitors that visit each site and observe what is being done during the study? There should be monitoring "Reports" that describe the results of all monitoring visits.

Costs and Resources

The third area we need to monitor to manage a clinical trial is the resources being used and their costs. It is not unusual for a study to start to run out of money before the trial is complete. We need to look at the reason for the cost overage. It can mean that things are being delayed or something is being done that isn't part of the study.

Perhaps the key to determining costs is what are the costs of the various resources required to do the work? Identifying resources and responsibilities is very important to managing the projects.

When planning and managing any job, one of the important things to work on is "Who is available to do the work and what work is each person supposed to do?" This is especially true for Clinical Trials because some of this information can impact Patient care and therefore their Safety.

Clinical Trials are typically "Sponsored" by a Pharmaceutical, Biotech, or Medical Device Company. They could also be sponsored by a University or other Research Center. There are also Contract Research Organizations (CROs) that will play the role of a sponsor to over-see the conduct of the research.

The actual study will be conducted by a Hospital or Clinic – a Site – where the patients will be seen for treatment.

Therefore we have the Sponsor who has the drug and is responsible for the research. This includes soliciting sites to see the patients and administer the drug. The number of sites will be determined by the number of patients required for the study, the drug and the illness being treated.

Project Management of Clinical Trials

It is worth mentioning that between the Sponsor and the Sites are "Monitors" whose job it is to make regular, frequent visits to the sites to assure that the study is being done in accordance with the study Protocol.

The study Protocol is a document that is critical to the study. It contains a detailed description of the drug, the treatment, the intended patient population, the study design, and more.

It should also be mentioned here that there is another group that will be visiting the sites. These are Quality Assurance Staff. The requirements for Quality Assurance will include monitoring of the sites. This will be accomplished by "independent" auditors who will also visit the sites and look for compliance or non-compliance to the protocol and applicable regulations.

Following are a set of "Roles" that will be used in this publication and used in the Excel Spreadsheets. However, the actual names of the roles can be changed very easily in the spreadsheets. So if, you have different "roles" for doing these tasks it will be easy to adopt the spreadsheets to your names.

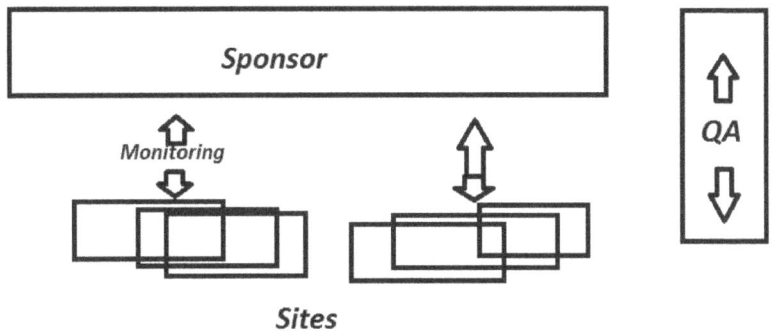

Typical Clinical Trial

There will be Roles and Responsibilities involving the following;

1. Sponsor

    The sponsor is responsible for the trial conduct and analysis.

2. Sites

    The sites will be responsible for conducting the study according to the direction set by the sponsor in the Protocol.

The Roles and Responsibilities of each can be as follows.

Sponsor

Role	Responsibility
Clinical	Must be responsible for all Medical aspects of the study. Over-sees preparation of the study Protocol and other Study Documentation.
Statistical	Prepares the Statistical Analysis Plan (SAP). Establishes the Study Design. Helps prepare all the data collection procedures and processes. This includes the CRF (Case Report Form), Randomization, and Sample Processing. Prepare the Statistical Analyses when the study is complete and contribute to the Clinical Summary.
Data Management	Prepares a Data Management Plan that describes the CRF or Data Entry procedures. It should also include any Data Clarification steps necessary to Lock the database.
Monitoring	Determine what will be checked on monitoring trips during the study. Schedule trips and necessary staff.

Project Management of Clinical Trials

Project Management	Develop a Plan for the study that tracks all key Dates, Resources, and Costs. Establish necessary funding. Hold regular meetings to track progress of the study and identify and help resolve any problems that might occur.
Quality Assurance	Conduct regular audits of all aspects of the study as the regulations require. Also conduct all QA Procedures required by the Company Quality Management System.
IT	Support all Computer aspects of the study.
Regulatory	Review all aspects of the study to assure that the study is being conducted in compliance with all relevant regulations.

Site

Role	Responsibility
Nurse Resource	A lot of the effort associated with seeing the patient and collecting the data is actually done by a Study Nurse.
Study Coordinator	It is usually good to have someone responsible for overseeing the details of the study conduct. This person is usually called a Study Coordinator. It may be the Study Nurse.
Principal Investigator	This is mainly the Investigator who is responsible for all aspects of the study at the site. They will see the patients and are responsible for the *contents* of the data and records collected.
Lab Effort	The processing of samples and specimens must be planned and then executed carefully to assure the results are entered and managed correctly.

Pharmacy	The Medications must be acquired with the proper labeling (blinding) and available when necessary for the patients. In some studies it is necessary to "account" for all medication.
IT	Support all Computer aspects of the study.
Accounting	It may be that the Finance or Accounting department will be involved in paying for supplies or billing the sponsor.
Other	There may be other resources that need to be estimated and tracked. This may be in the form of other instrumentation or diagnostic tools.

There is nothing magical about the names of these resources. If necessary, you will be able to substitute other names for these resources.

We recommend not getting more detailed. For example, you can obviously put the names of specific people in here. We recommend against that. The planning and managing being discussed here is best done at a level where the numbers and dates can be reviewed and updated if need be. What you don't want to do is change names as people change. If one of the resources leaves the company or is reassigned or promoted, you don't want to always be updating the plan.

If the plan is too detailed it can be a major task to update and the plan will become an end instead of a means to an end.

6. Planning a Trial

In most cases a clinical trial has three parts;

- Study Start up – Preparing the site and identifying potential patients
- Study Execution – The period from the first patient visit to the last patient visit
- Study Close out – The period after the visits when the database is finalized and the analyses and summaries are prepared.

1. Study Start-up

    The activities associated with starting a study are the following;

    Study Protocol – A Study protocol is a document that describes in detail the design and operation of the study. This document is prepared by the sponsor and should cover virtually all aspects of the trial. This document needs to be approved and signed-off before the patients are seen.

    IRB Approval – Each study site usually has an Institutional Review Board (IRB) that over sees the research done at the site. The IRB has to approve conduct of the study at that site.

Setup Data Collection and Entry – Data entry is typically done either by paper CRFs entered into a computer or entered directly into the computer during the patient visit.

Identify Potential Patients and Begin Scheduling Visits – The site will want to identify the patients for the study and begin to develop schedules for patient visits. This may involve doing some advertising or other activity to identify people interested in the study.

Arrange for Processing of Fluid Samples, Urine, Blood, etc. – The processing of study samples may involve special containers to ship samples that need to be frozen.

Arrange for Medication – Work with the sponsor to insure study medications are available when the patients visit. The medications may require special labels or other packaging.

The study Start-up ends with the first patient visit.

2. Study Execution

The study execution step goes on as long as patients are coming in for visits. The activities during this step would be;

Conducting patient visits – The patients will come in and be observed as is called for in the protocol. This typically will involve the study nurse see the patient first and record some basic information. On the first visit, the biggest issue may be the inclusion/exclusion criteria for the study. After the basic information is collected, the investigator will see the patient and review the information recorded.

for accuracy. Then they will continue to record the heavier medical information.

Collection of Necessary Samples and Specimens – This should be described in detail in the study protocol. These activities will be monitored and checked by QA during the study.

Distribution of Study Medication – This is obviously a very important step and in cases where it is a new type of medication there can be specific government regulations that need to be followed.

3. Study Close-out

    The goals are to

- complete any Patient follow-up
- complete and "lock" the database
- run all Statistical Analyses
- prepare the Clinical Summary(s)
- archive all necessary records.

Some of these activities will be shared between the sponsor and the site. For example, all study documentation (records) from the site and from the sponsor and will need to be archived for a specific retention period in a format that allows for quick retrieval during an audit or inspection.

In some cases blood samples are taken and may need to be stored (frozen) for later analyses. Many companies now are taking genetic samples that can be analyzed at a later date.

6.1 *Estimation of Study Dates, Resources, and Costs*

Obviously a big part of planning will be estimating the Dates, Resources, and costs. We will do this estimating at three levels;

1. Defaults

   The first level assumes that there is some information that will be the same regardless of the study such as the rates charged for some of the resources.

2. Standard Studies

   The second level is to develop a set of "Standard" studies. There might be estimates that can be used for a "standard" Phase I trial or a trial for one division of the hospital.

3. Individual Studies

   Finally, each study will have a set of estimates for the dates, resources, and costs.

When assembling the plan, the first step is developing a list of the studies. Each study is then matched with the "Standard" study, looking for similarities to the study in the plan.

Make a copy of the spreadsheet that most closely matches the study and rename the spreadsheet by changing the name on the tab for the spreadsheet.

The spreadsheet will be populated with estimates either from the Default values or from the Standard Study spreadsheet. The final step for this study is to review the estimates for possible use in the plan. If not used, the estimates can be changed.

The estimates will typically come from one of three sources;

1. The values in the Defaults or the Standard studies

2. Values that you based on experience or other knowledge

3. They can be calculated from different study parameters

    Values such as the number of patients, the number of pages in the CRF, or the number of visits/month can sometimes be used to develop estimates for the dates or required resources.

    For example, if you know it takes 15 minutes for a nurse to see a patient per page of a CRF and the study you have has 8 pages in the CRF, then each visit will take two hours of a nurse's time. If there are 20 patient visits per month that means 40 hours per month for the nurse or one-quarter time or .25 per month.

    There is an area on the spreadsheets for studies to do these calculations.

The costs for the various resources are entered on a monthly rate. The total costs will be based on the dates and the amount of the resource estimated.

The estimates for the dates are fairly simple. If we assume there are three parts to each study we need to estimate four values. These are;

1. The Start date for the "Study Start-up"
2. The number of days the Study Start-up will take
3. The number of days the Study Execution will last
4. The number of days the Study Close-out will take.

Project Management of Clinical Trials

For planning purposes the Defaults assume that the Study Start-up and the Study Close-out will each take 3 months. The study start date and the duration of the Study Execution will obviously depend on the study.

The tables that follow contain values for estimates for the effort required for these resources and the associated costs. It should be emphasized that these values are simply "plug" numbers. Your numbers might be very different.

If the study is very similar to other studies that you have conducted the numbers might be much smaller. It should take fewer resources to do the study. If the study is for a new drug and the study has a large number of patients then these numbers might be too small.

Another point to consider is if you are preparing an annual budget this Excel spreadsheet might be very helpful. It can be very helpful to do some "sensitivity analyses". That is, you can ask the question, "What if the study doesn't finish in May but is delayed until November. It would be very easy to go in and change the dates and obtain new cost estimates.

The "organization" for a clinical trial is usually simple. The investigator is responsible for all aspects of the study. This is to a large degree because of their medical training. It is also because the FDA regulations state this. There will also be a nursing staff that helps to see and treat the patients. Generally one of the nurses will fulfill the role of a study "Coordinator". They will usually handle a lot of the administrative tasks associated with the study. This can include managing the documents and other records, scheduling patients, tracking samples, managing the medications, and reporting any issues.

The Pharmacy will usually be responsible for stocking, storage, and distribution of the study medications.

Project Management of Clinical Trials

The Central Lab will be responsible for accepting the study samples, producing the necessary analyses, storing the samples, and returning the results to the study site.

Of course there can be other groups involved in the study. For example, a diagnostic lab that does X-rays or MRIs may be a valued resource.

Following are some tables that show the various Roles, the Responsibilities of each Role and then give a "potential" estimate of the amount of that resource. The amount of resource will vary considerably from study to study. You need to consider the study and then be able to estimate the amount of that resource required.

There are tables for each part of a clinical trial – Study Start, Study Execution, and Study Close-out. In each of these three areas there are two tables, one for the Sponsor and one for the Site.

Sponsor

Role	Responsibility	Amount
Clinical	Must be responsible for all Medical aspects of the study. Over-sees preparation of the study Protocol and other Study Documentation.	.75 = Three quarter to almost full time
Statistical	Prepare the Study Design and Data Collection portion of the Study Protocol Assist the preparation of the CRF Prepare the Statistical Analysis Plan.	.25 = One-quarter time
Data Management	Prepare a Data Management Plan Prepare the study CRF Help to prepare Data Edit checks	.5 = Half-time to prepare the CRF and setup data entry

Project Management of Clinical Trials

Monitoring	Plan the Monitoring trips to the Sites during the study	.25 = One-quarter time
Project Management	Develop written plans with dates, necessary resources, and associated costs.	.25 = One-quarter time
Quality Assurance	Prepare a QA Plan of activities to be performed during the trial	.1 = One-tenth time
IT	Prepare or assist with preparation of any software needed during the trial. This could include the Data Entry system, any Laboratory systems,	.5 = Half-time to setup the Data Entry procedures and equipment
Regulatory	Review the study operations for compliance.	.25 = One-quarter time to review study documents
Accounting	Prepare and execute budgeting	.10 = One-tenth time to pay bills

Department - Personnel	Effort/Month	Mo. Rate ($k)
Clinical	.75	15.00
Statistical	.25	10.00
Data Management	.5	5.00
Monitoring	.25	8.00
Project Management	.25	8.00
Quality Assurance	.1	5.00
IT	.5	5.00
Regulatory	.25	8.00
Accounting	.1	5.00
Other Monthly Costs		
Drug Supplies	2.0	
Lab Processing	0.0	

Site

Role	Responsibility	Amount
Nurse Resource	Make any preparations for the visits Begin to Schedule Patients	.75 = Three-quarter time
Study Coordinator	Someone responsible for overseeing the details of the study conduct. They may be the Study Nurse.	1.0 = One full-time person
Investigator	Prepare the site for the study Assist with getting IRB Approval	.5 = One-half time for the Investigator.
Lab Effort	Prepare to Process Sample and Report Results	.25 = One-quarter time
Pharmacy	Stock necessary medication	.25 = One-Quarter time
IT	Prepare or assist with preparation of any software needed during the trial. This could include the Data Entry system, any Laboratory systems,	.1 = One-tenth time.
Accounting	Take care of any billing or paying of bills necessary	.1 = One-tenth
Other		

Department - Personnel	Effort/Month	Mo. Rate ($k)
Nurse Resource	1.00	5.00
Study Coordinator	1.00	7.00
Investigator	2.00	15.00
Lab Effort	1.00	10.00
Pharmacy	0.50	10.00
IT	0.50	5.00
Accounting	0.10	5.00
Other		
Other Monthly Costs		
Drug Supplies		
Lab Processing		

Study Execution

The goal during study execution is to monitor the safety of the patient and;

- see the patients according to the schedule in the protocol
- collect the required information in an accurate way
- administer the medication according to the protocol
- monitor the activities to see they are being done correctly
- conduct periodic audits of the study

During the study execution, most effort goes on at the sites rather than at the sponsor. In a very large study the hospital or clinic may dedicate full-time staff and part of a building wing to seeing the study patients.

Sponsor

Role	Responsibility	Amount
Clinical	The medical staff at the sponsor will largely monitor progress and answer questions. There may be Investigator meetings they would attend.	.1 = one-tenth time for the medical staff
Statistical	The statistician will generally monitor progress during the study.	.1 = one-tenth for the statistician
Data Management	The role of the data manager will depend on how the data is entered. If paper CRFS are used then they will have data entry to perform. If electronic data capture (EDC) is used then their role will be more one of monitoring progress.	.5 = half-time for the data manager
Monitoring	The monitor will schedule visits to each site. The frequency and length will be based on the type of study and the number of patients at each site.	1.0 – full-time for the study monitor

Project Management of Clinical Trials

Project Management	The Project Management department will also track study progress and look for issues. They will also typically be involved in budgeting for the study.	.25 = one-quarter time
Quality Assurance	QA should schedule audits to a sampling of some of the sites.	.1 = one-tenth
IT	Support the computer aspects of the study. Their role and amount of effort will also depend on the data entry method – Paper CRF or EDC.	.25 = one-quarter time
Regulatory	The regulatory affairs department will monitor study activities to assure all regulatory aspects of the study are in compliance.	.1 = one-tenth time
Accounting	Prepare and execute budgeting	.10 = One-tenth time to pay bills

Department - Personnel	Effort/Month	Mo. Rate ($k)
Clinical	.1	15.00
Statistical	.1	10.00
Data Management	.5	5.00
Monitoring	1.0	8.00
Project Management	.25	8.00
Quality Assurance	.1	5.00
IT	.25	5.00
Regulatory	.1	8.00
Accounting	.1	5.00
Other Monthly Costs		
Drug Supplies	2.0	
Lab Processing	1.0	

Site

Role	Responsibility	Amount
Nurse Resource	See the patients and make some observations. Prepare the patient to see the Investigator, and take necessary samples.	1.00
Study Coordinator	Schedule patients, make sure the data is accurately recorded. Track any records for the study.	1.00
Investigator	See the patients, record the necessary data, and administer the medications based on the protocol.	1.00
Lab Effort	Analyze the samples from the study and report the results.	1.00
Pharmacy	Distribute the medications in accordance with the protocol	0.50
IT	Assist with any data collection.	0.50
Accounting	Take care of any billing or paying of bills necessary	.1 = One-tenth
Other		

Department - Personnel	Effort/Month	Mo. Rate ($k)
Nurse Resource	1.00	5.00
Study Coordinator	1.00	7.00
Investigator	1.00	15.00
Lab Effort	1.00	10.00
Pharmacy	0.50	10.00
IT	0.50	5.00
Accounting	0.10	5.00
Other		
Other Monthly Costs		
Drug Supplies		
Lab Processing		

Study Close-out

Sponsor

Role	Responsibility	Amount
Clinical	Review study conduct for compliance to protocol. Complete Clinical Summary.	.75
Statistical	Review Database content and do the necessary statistical analysis. Contribute to Clinical Summary.	.25
Data Management	Complete the lock of the database and assemble all data documentation.	.5
Monitoring	Summarize monitoring visits	.1
Project Management	Document study progress. Prepare any budgeting necessary to complete the study	.25
Quality Assurance	Review all Quality aspects to the study. Conduct any audits or other steps necessary to make a quality statement regarding the study	.1
IT	Help to finish the study database and the archival of all electronic records.	.5
Regulatory	Review the storage and retrieval of all study records and data	.25
Accounting	Prepare and execute budgeting	.10 = One-tenth time to pay bills

Department - Personnel	Effort/Month	Mo. Rate ($k)
Clinical	.75	15.00
Statistical	.25	10.00
Data Management	.5	5.00
Monitoring	.25	8.00
Project Management	.25	8.00
Quality Assurance	.1	5.00

IT	.5	5.00
Regulatory	.25	8.00
Accounting	.1	5.00
Other Monthly Costs		
Drug Supplies	2.0	
Lab Processing	0.0	

Site

Role	Responsibility	Amount
Nurse Resource	Complete all data necessary for the study. Provide all study records for archival.	1.0
Study Coordinator	Document the completion of all aspects of the study at the site.	0.5
Investigator	Finalize and sign all study records. Review the Statistical analyses and Clinical Summaries.	0.5
Lab Effort	Complete all sample analyses. Store any samples that need long-term storage.	0.2
Pharmacy	Account for any Medication not used in the study	0.2
IT	Assist the completion of the study database. Assist with the return of any equipment.	0.1

Department - Personnel	Effort/Month	Mo. Rate ($k)
Nurse Resource	1.0	5.00
Study Coordinator	0.5	7.00
Investigator	0.5	15.00
Lab Effort	0.2	10.00
Pharmacy	0.2	10.00
IT	0.1	5.00

Project Management of Clinical Trials

Other Monthly Costs		
Drug Supplies		
Lab Processing		

Assembling the three steps together we use the following table to generate the resource and cost estimates.

Sponsor

Department - Personnel	Start-up	Execution	Close-out	Mo. Rate ($k)
Clinical	1.00	1.00	2.00	5.00
Statistical	1.00	0.50	2.00	10.00
Data Management	2.00	2.00	1.00	15.00
Monitoring	1.00	0.50	1.00	12.00
Project Management	0.50	0.50	0.50	10.00
Quality Assurance	0.50	0.10	0.10	5.00
IT				
Regulatory				
Other Monthly Costs				
Drug Supplies	2.0	5.0	0.0	
Lab Processing	0.0	2.0	0.0	
Annual Fixed Costs		Month	Amount ($k)	
Other Computer		6.0	10.0	
Other Computer		7.0	2.0	
Other Personnel		8.0	3.0	
Other Procedures		9.0	4.0	

Site

Department - Personnel	Start-up	Execution	Close-out	Mo. Rate ($k)
Nurse Resource	1.00	1.00	2.00	5.00
Study Coordinator	1.00	0.50	2.00	7.00
Investigator	2.00	2.00	1.00	15.00
Lab Effort	1.00	0.50	1.00	10.00
Pharmacy	0.50	0.50	0.50	10.00
IT	0.50	0.10	0.10	5.00
Accounting	0.10	0.10	0.10	5.00
Other				
Department - Personnel	**Start-up**	**Execution**	**Close-out**	**Mo. Rate ($k)**
Other Monthly Costs				
Drug Supplies	2.0	5.0	0.0	
Lab Processing	0.0	2.0	0.0	
Annual Fixed Costs		**Month**	**Amount ($k)**	
Other Computer		6.0	10.0	
Other Computer		7.0	2.0	
Other Personnel		8.0	3.0	
Other Procedures		9.0	4.0	

If we know the start and stop dates for the three steps we can calculate the amount of resources required and the associated costs for either the Sponsor or the Site.

If, for example, the dates were;

Study Start-up	6/1/2017	8/31/2017	3 mo.
Study Execution	9/1/2017	4/30/2018	8 mo.
Study Close-out	5/1/2018	7/31/2018	3 mo.

– Notes –

As these numbers are reported are they larger or smaller than expected. Either way it can indicate a potential problem. Are all of the required resources reporting time?

It can be difficult in some of these cases to collect "actual" time. Many medical clinics and hospitals do not report time. It might be necessary to just assume that whatever was planned was what was used.

7. Estimating Costs and Resources using Excel

To implement the Project Management principles it will likely be necessary to use a computer system. There are a variety of such systems that could be used. You need to review the options that would work best for your studies, your staffs, and other requirements of your organization. The examples here used Microsoft Excel and the spreadsheet files are available for you to use and modify if necessary.

7.1 Use Excel or MS Project

- Resource Costs
- Amount of Effort required for each Resource at each Step
- Calculate Budget by Multiplying Cost x effort x Time.

Microsoft Project will do much of the same thing but it tends to "anticipate" some values differently than what is needed. However, I recommend that you look at both systems and see which works best for you, your studies, and your organization.

Project Management of Clinical Trials

7.2 An Example with Excel

- Build a "System" for a set of Trials (Portfolio?)
  - Default Values – Typically do not change from one trial to another
    - Hourly Charges
    - Time to produce an analysis
  - Typical or Sample Studies – by drug, by Phase, by Drug type
  - From These Generate One Spreadsheet for each Real Study
  - Spreadsheets to Display Monthly/Annual Totals

Enter "Actuals" if Possible

7.3 "Default Values"

Plan Start 1-Jan-19		Organization Name					
	Length of Start up	Length of Execution	Length of Close				
	90	N/A	90	Mo. Rate			
Department - Personnel		Effort/Month		($k)	Units		Description
Nurse Resource	1.00	1.00	2.00	5.00	Resources		Effort/Month E.g. .5 means 1/5 person for 1 month
Study Coordinator	1.00	0.50	2.00	10.00			If the effort is 10 days/month that is about .25.
Investigator	2.00	2.00	1.00	15.00			
Lab Effort	1.00	0.50	1.00	12.00	Mo. Rate		The amount that the resources will cost for 1 month.
Pharmacy	0.50	0.50	0.50	10.00	Length of Start-up		Number of Days
IT	0.50	0.10	0.10	5.00	Length of Close		Number of Days
Accounting	0.20	0.10	0.20	5.00			
Other	0.00	0.00	0.00	0.00			
					Length of Study Execution		Number of Days
Other Monthly Costs							
Drug Supplies	2.0	5.0	0.0				
Lab Processing	0.0	2.0	0.0				
Annual Fixed Costs		Month	Amount ($k)				
Other Computer		6.0	10.0				
Other Computer		7.0	2.0				
Other Personnel		8.0	3.0				
Other Procedures		9.0	4.0				

Entries are used to calculate DATES
Entries are used to calculate the amount and cost of RESOURCES

Project Management of Clinical Trials

7.4 Study Effort

	Length of Study Execution		Study Start	Start Execution	Last Patient Visit	Summary Complete				
Study Start										
3/1/2017	120		1-Mar-17	30-May-17	27-Sep-17	26-Dec-17				
No. Patients & Sites	30	4	Monthly Personnel Requirements				Total Personnel Cost ($k)			
Department - Personnel			Study Start	Execution	Close out	Monthly Cost ($k)	Study Start	Execution	Close out	Total Costs
Nurse Resource			1.0	1.0	2.0	5.0	15.0	20.0	30.0	65
Study Coordinator			1.0	0.5	2.0	10.0	30.0	20.0	60.0	110
Investigator			2.0	2.0	1.0	15.0	90.0	120.0	45.0	255
Lab Effort			1.0	0.5	1.0	12.0	36.0	24.0	36.0	96
Pharmacy			0.5	0.5	0.5	10.0	15.0	20.0	15.0	50
IT			0.5	0.1	0.1	5.0	7.5	2.0	1.5	11
Accounting			0.2	0.1	0.2	5.0	3.0	2.0	3.0	8
Other			0.0	0.0	0.0	0.0	0.0	0.0	0.0	0
Other Monthly Costs										
Drug Supplies			2	5	0		6	20	0	26
Lab Processing			0	2	0		0	8	0	8
Annual Fixed Costs			Month	Amount						
Other Computer			6	10						10
Other Computer			7	2						2
Other Personnel			8	3						3
Other Procedures			9	4						4
Total										648

7.5 Execute and Control the Clinical Plans

- Plans are "Alive"
- Focus First on Deliverables
    - Regulations
    - Responsibilities
    - Compliance
    - Quality
- Data Quality and Integrity

Project Management of Clinical Trials

Execute and Control the Clinical Plans
Total Projections

Study Title		Group IV - Last Drug Trial							
Protocol #	PR001234								
Drug(s)	Cure-all 01								
Study Phase	Phase III								
Description									

	Study Start	Length of Study Execution	Study Start	Start Execution	Last Patient Visit	Summary Complete			
	11/1/2019	60	1-Nov-19	30-Jan-20	30-Mar-20	28-Jun-20			
No. Patients & Sites	30	4	Monthly Personnel Requirements				Total Personnel Cost ($k)		

Department - Personnel	Study Start	Execution	Close out	Monthly Cost ($k)	Study Start	Execution	Close out	Total Costs
Nurse Resource	1.0	1.0	2.0	5.0	15.0	10.0	30.0	55
Study Coordinator	1.0	0.5	2.0	10.0	30.0	10.0	60.0	100
Investigator	2.0	2.0	1.0	15.0	90.0	60.0	45.0	195
Lab Effort	1.0	0.5	1.0	12.0	36.0	12.0	36.0	84
Pharmacy	0.5	0.5	0.5	10.0	15.0	10.0	15.0	40
IT	0.5	0.1	0.1	5.0	7.5	1.0	1.5	10
Accounting	0.2	0.1	0.2	5.0	3.0	1.0	3.0	7
Other	0.0	0.0	0.0	0.0	0.0	0.0	0.0	0
Other Monthly Costs								
Drug Supplies	2	5	0		6	10	0	16
Lab Processing	0	2	0		0	4	0	4
Annual Fixed Costs	Month	Amount						
Other Computer	6	10						10
Other Computer	7	2						2
Other Personnel	8	3						3
Other Procedures	9	4						4
Total								530

7.6 Start-up Resources

Review the Monthly Resources
- Are there enough – In General
- Are there too many – In General
- Are they the correct Resources

Are there any potential Problem Areas?

Project Management of Clinical Trials

7.7 Gantt Chart

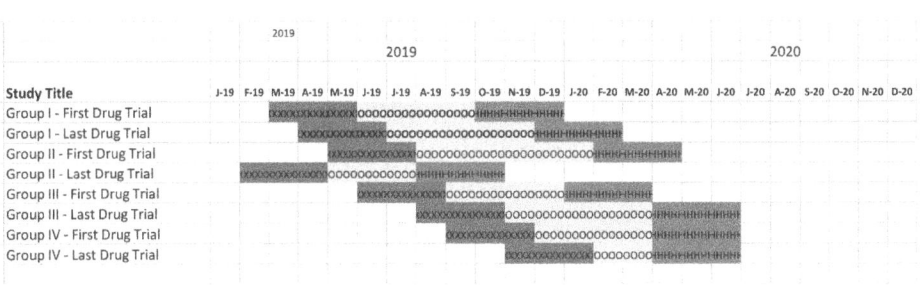

7.8 Execute and Control the Clinical Plans Monthly Projections

Total Resource Costs ($k)

	2019					2020				
	Group I	Group II	Group III	Group IV	Total	Group I	Group II	Group III	Group IV	Total
Department - Personnel										
Nurse Resource	114.4	99.3	60.6	30.0	304.4	18.6	33.7	67.8	79.3	199.4
Study Coordinator	184.6	158.7	91.4	54.8	489.6	37.1	63.4	125.8	143.3	369.6
Investigator	503.1	464.1	358.1	180.0	1,505.2	27.9	68.7	145.7	209.2	451.5
Lab Effort	172.7	155.2	108.2	65.8	501.9	22.3	40.5	81.4	100.8	244.9
Pharmacy	94.0	84.7	60.0	30.0	268.7	9.3	18.9	38.8	49.7	116.6
IT	21.2	20.5	17.8	12.9	72.4	0.9	1.9	3.9	6.8	13.5
Accounting	14.4	12.9	9.0	5.5	41.8	1.9	3.4	6.8	8.4	20.4
Other	0.0	0.0	0.0	0.0	0.0	0.0	0.0	0.0	0.0	0.0
Other Monthly Costs										
Drug Supplies	57.0	52.0	42.0	15.0	166.0	0.0	5.0	15.0	27.0	47.0
Lab Processing	18.0	16.0	12.0	2.0	48.0	0.0	2.0	6.0	10.0	18.0
Annual Fixed Costs										
Other Computer	20.0	20.0	0.0	0.0	40.0	0.0	0.0	10.0	20.0	30.0
Other Computer	4.0	4.0	2.0	0.0	10.0	0.0	0.0	0.0	0.0	0.0
Other Personnel	6.0	6.0	3.0	0.0	15.0	0.0	0.0	0.0	0.0	0.0
Other Procedures	8.0	8.0	8.0	0.0	24.0	0.0	0.0	0.0	0.0	0.0
Total	1,217.5		772.2		3,487.0					

Department - Personnel	Jan-19	Feb-19	Mar-19	Apr-19	May-19	Jun-19	Jul-19	Aug-19	Sep-19	Oct-19	Nov-19	Dec-19	Total Person Months	Total Person Costs ($k)
Nurse Resource	0.0	0.0	0.0	0.0	0.0	0.0	0.0	0.0	0.0	0.0	1.0	1.0	2.0	10.0
Study Coordinator	0.0	0.0	0.0	0.0	0.0	0.0	0.0	0.0	0.0	0.0	1.0	1.0	2.0	20.0
Investigator	0.0	0.0	0.0	0.0	0.0	0.0	0.0	0.0	0.0	0.0	2.0	2.0	4.0	60.0
Lab Effort	0.0	0.0	0.0	0.0	0.0	0.0	0.0	0.0	0.0	0.0	1.0	1.0	2.0	24.0
Pharmacy	0.0	0.0	0.0	0.0	0.0	0.0	0.0	0.0	0.0	0.0	0.5	0.5	1.0	10.0
IT	0.0	0.0	0.0	0.0	0.0	0.0	0.0	0.0	0.0	0.0	0.5	0.5	1.0	5.0
Accounting	0.0	0.0	0.0	0.0	0.0	0.0	0.0	0.0	0.0	0.0	0.2	0.2	0.4	2.0
Other	0.0	0.0	0.0	0.0	0.0	0.0	0.0	0.0	0.0	0.0	0.0	0.0	0.0	0.0
Other Monthly Costs														
Drug Supplies	0.0	0.0	0.0	0.0	0.0	0.0	0.0	0.0	0.0	0.0	2.0	2.0		4.0
Lab Processing	0.0	0.0	0.0	0.0	0.0	0.0	0.0	0.0	0.0	0.0	0.0	0.0		0.0
Annual Fixed Costs														
Other Computer	0.0	0.0	0.0	0.0	0.0	0.0	0.0	0.0	0.0	0.0	0.0	0.0		0.0
Other Computer	0.0	0.0	0.0	0.0	0.0	0.0	0.0	0.0	0.0	0.0	0.0	0.0		0.0
Other Personnel	0.0	0.0	0.0	0.0	0.0	0.0	0.0	0.0	0.0	0.0	0.0	0.0		0.0
Other Procedures	0.0	0.0	0.0	0.0	0.0	0.0	0.0	0.0	0.0	0.0	0.0	0.0		0.0
Total	0.0	0.0	0.0	0.0	0.0	0.0	0.0	0.0	0.0	0.0	8.2	8.2		135.0

Execute and Control the Clinical Plans
Monthly Projections

- Can you get "Actuals"?
- Has anything forced a Change?
    - Drug Safety Monitoring Committee?
    - End Point Study?
- A Change in Patient Enrollment?
- New Adverse Events?

- Monitoring Reports
    - Patient Enrollment Rate
    - Data Error Rates
    - Data "Questions"
    - Timeliness of Laboratory Reporting
    - Unexpected Drop-outs
- Periodic Site Audits

Close the Project

- Finish the Deliverables (Signed-off, and Dated)
    - Reports
    - Files
    - Archives
- Reports
    - Begin Programming Reports before study is complete?
        - Build SAS Datasets
        - Write SAS Programs
    - Have Reports ready to run day of Last Patient/Last Visit

- Pay Remaining Expenses
    - Salaries
    - CROs
    - Labs
- Dispose of Remaining Medication?

Project Management of Clinical Trials

- Was the Project Done Right?
- Was it the Best? Is there a Better Way?
- Quality

Key Ingredients

- Documented Evidence
- Process (Procedures)
- Perform (Proof)
- Consistently
- Quality Attributes (Was it done Right?)
- Specifications (What and How)
- <u>All Necessary for Quality Management, Risk Management, Validation, Qualification, Compliance, and Others</u>

Summary Topics

- Define clinical project management
- Plan the work
- Produce the schedule
- Estimate Dates
- Work in teams
- Forecast a clinical trial budget
- Execute and control the clinical plans
- Close the project

--Notes --

8. The Excel Worksheets

Defaults

The values we have presented thus far are entered in the "Defaults" spreadsheet. The assumption would be that these values will be similar for all of our studies. For a Site the Defaults spreadsheet would contain the following;

Project Management of Clinical Trials

	Plan Start 1-Jan-19				
		\multicolumn{3}{c}{Organization Name}		
		Length of Start up	Length of Execution	Length of Close	
		90	N/A	90	
Department - Personnel		\multicolumn{3}{c}{Effort/Month}		Mo. Rate ($k)
Nurse Resource		1.00	1.00	2.00	5.00
Study Coordinator		1.00	0.50	2.00	10.00
Investigator		2.00	2.00	1.00	15.00
Lab Effort		1.00	0.50	1.00	12.00
Pharmacy		0.50	0.50	0.50	10.00
IT		0.50	0.10	0.10	5.00
Accounting		0.20	0.10	0.20	5.00
Other		0.00	0.00	0.00	0.00
Other Monthly Costs					
Drug Supplies		2.0	5.0	0.0	
Lab Processing		0.0	2.0	0.0	
Annual Fixed Costs			Month	Amount ($k)	
Other Computer			6.0	10.0	
Other Computer			7.0	2.0	
Other Personnel			8.0	3.0	
Other Procedures			9.0	4.0	

Entries are used to calculate DATES
Entries are used to calculate the amount and cost of RESOURCES

All of the shaded cells can be changed and they will be reflected throughout the other spreadsheets. These values are automatically copied to the spreadsheets that follow.

Having said this, the values that follow in the subsequent spreadsheets can be changed and then those values will be reflected in the spreadsheets that follow those.

The same is true for the Files used for the Sponsor.

Each of the Excel files start with a single Defaults Spreadsheet. Following this spreadsheet is a set of spreadsheets, one spreadsheet for each Standard type of study. For example, there might be four standard spreadsheets, one for Phase I studies, one for Phase II studies, one for Phase III studies, and one for Phase IV studies.

Project Management of Clinical Trials

The first Default Study spreadsheet in the file begins with the following;

Study Title				Drug I Trial						
Protocol #										
Drug(s)										
Study Phase										
Description										
		Length of Study Execution		Start	Last Patient Visit	Summary Complete				
Study Start			Study Start	Execution						
3/1/2019		120	1-Mar-19	30-May-19	27-Sep-19	26-Dec-19				
No. Patients & Sites		30	4	Monthly Personnel Requirements			Total Personnel Cost ($k)			
Department - Personnel			Study Start	Execution	Close out	Monthly Cost ($k)	Study Start	Execution	Close out	Total Costs
Nurse Resource			1.0	1.0	2.0	5.0	15.0	20.0	30.0	65
Study Coordinator			1.0	0.5	2.0	10.0	30.0	20.0	60.0	110
Investigator			2.0	2.0	1.0	15.0	90.0	120.0	45.0	255
Lab Effort			1.0	0.5	1.0	12.0	36.0	24.0	36.0	96
Pharmacy			0.5	0.5	0.5	10.0	15.0	20.0	15.0	50
IT			0.5	0.1	0.1	5.0	7.5	2.0	1.5	11
Accounting			0.2	0.1	0.2	5.0	3.0	2.0	3.0	8
Other			0.0	0.0	0.0	0.0	0.0	0.0	0.0	0
Other Monthly Costs										
Drug Supplies			2	5	0		6	20	0	26
Lab Processing			0	2	0		0	8	0	8
Annual Fixed Costs			Month	Amount						
Other Computer			6	10						10
Other Computer			7	2						2
Other Personnel			8	3						3
Other Procedures			9	4						4
Total										648
				Alternative Method of Estimation of Monthly Resources for this Study						
Other Parameters							Study Start	Execution	Close out	Person Monthly Cost ($k)
Number of Visits			10		Nurse Resource					
Number of Sites			5		Study Coordinator					
Length of study - Mo.			6		Investigator					
No. Pages in CRF			12		Lab Effort					
Study Phase			1		Pharmacy					
No. Monitoring trips/Mo										
Special Equipment										

The cells shaded *gray* at the top of the page are descriptive study information. This information is "carried" forward onto the specific study spreadsheets. None of this information is used for calculations.

Below this are two cells shaded *green*. These entries are used to calculate the dates. The cells that are shaded *blue* are used to calculate an estimated resource if that is necessary.

Near the bottom is a section of cells shaded *yellow*. These can be used to estimate the amount of resources (or dates) required.

The part of the spreadsheet to the right of the Resource Estimates will show the total costs for the study. These figures should be usable for any budgeting necessary.

To the right of this part of the spreadsheet are two tables; one for each of the next two years showing the resource costs by month for that study.

Department - Personnel	Jan-19	Feb-19	Mar-19	Apr-19	May-19	Jun-19	Jul-19	Aug-19	Sep-19	Oct-19	Nov-19	Dec-19	Total Person Months	Total Person Costs ($k)
Nurse Resource	0.0	0.0	0.0	0.0	0.0	0.0	0.0	0.0	0.0	0.0	1.0	1.0	2.0	10.0
Study Coordinator	0.0	0.0	0.0	0.0	0.0	0.0	0.0	0.0	0.0	0.0	1.0	1.0	2.0	20.0
Investigator	0.0	0.0	0.0	0.0	0.0	0.0	0.0	0.0	0.0	0.0	2.0	2.0	4.0	60.0
Lab Effort	0.0	0.0	0.0	0.0	0.0	0.0	0.0	0.0	0.0	0.0	1.0	1.0	2.0	24.0
Pharmacy	0.0	0.0	0.0	0.0	0.0	0.0	0.0	0.0	0.0	0.0	0.5	0.5	1.0	10.0
IT	0.0	0.0	0.0	0.0	0.0	0.0	0.0	0.0	0.0	0.0	0.5	0.5	1.0	5.0
Accounting	0.0	0.0	0.0	0.0	0.0	0.0	0.0	0.0	0.0	0.0	0.2	0.2	0.4	2.0
Other	0.0	0.0	0.0	0.0	0.0	0.0	0.0	0.0	0.0	0.0	0.0	0.0	0.0	0.0
Other Monthly Costs														
Drug Supplies	0.0	0.0	0.0	0.0	0.0	0.0	0.0	0.0	0.0	0.0	2.0	2.0		4.0
Lab Processing	0.0	0.0	0.0	0.0	0.0	0.0	0.0	0.0	0.0	0.0	0.0	0.0		0.0
Annual Fixed Costs														
Other Computer	0.0	0.0	0.0	0.0	0.0	0.0	0.0	0.0	0.0	0.0	0.0	0.0		0.0
Other Computer	0.0	0.0	0.0	0.0	0.0	0.0	0.0	0.0	0.0	0.0	0.0	0.0		0.0
Other Personnel	0.0	0.0	0.0	0.0	0.0	0.0	0.0	0.0	0.0	0.0	0.0	0.0		0.0
Other Procedures	0.0	0.0	0.0	0.0	0.0	0.0	0.0	0.0	0.0	0.0	0.0	0.0		0.0
Total	0.0	0.0	0.0	0.0	0.0	0.0	0.0	0.0	0.0	0.0	8.2	8.2		135.0

There should be a spreadsheet like this for each "type" of trail conducted. As was mentioned above, there might be one spreadsheet for the type of study – Phase I through Phase IV.

It might be good to have one (or two or three) spreadsheets for each drug being studied, but the idea is that these "standard" studies form the basis or building block for the Plan.

To get the set of standard studies for your organization, make copies of these spreadsheets and modify the entries where necessary to reflect the values in those standard studies.

Developing the Plan

To actually develop the plan, begin with a list of the studies needed in the plan. Each study is then matched with a "Standard"

Project Management of Clinical Trials

study, looking for similarities to the actual study in the plan. When you have the list of "Standard" studies similar to each of the actual studies, copy those "standard" study spreadsheets to a spreadsheet for the matching actual study.

Then go into each spreadsheet and make the necessary adjustments to reflect the details of that study.

When the spreadsheets are copied, all spreadsheets for a given drug or given study Phase should be grouped together. Some "Summaries" that follow will "group" the information in the spreadsheets to produce totals for the drug across all of the studies.

Study Summaries

Once all of the studies are defined in the plan, there will be some summaries that display information across all of the studies.

Perhaps the simplest display is the Gantt Chart of Studies.

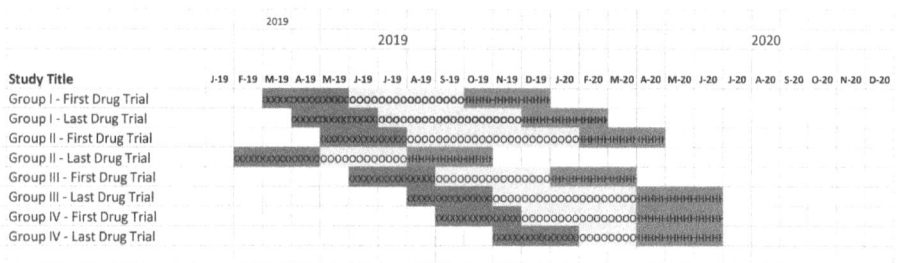

Another summary is below

The following summary will show the total costs by study by year across all resources.

	Study Title	No. of Patients	Study Start	Execution Start	Study Completion	Clinical Summary	Total Cost ($k) 2019	2020
GroupITrialA	Group I - First Drug Trial	30	1-Mar-19	30-May-19	27-Sep-19	26-Dec-19	636.4	0.0
GroupITrialX	Group I - Last Drug Trial	30	1-Apr-19	30-Jun-19	27-Nov-19	25-Feb-20	581.1	117.9
GroupIITrialA	Group II - First Drug Trial	30	1-May-19	30-Jul-19	26-Jan-20	25-Apr-20	518.2	237.4
GroupIITrialX	Group II - Last Drug Trial	30	5-Jan-19	5-Apr-19	4-Jul-19	2-Oct-19	583.2	0.0
GroupIIITrialA	Group III - First Drug Trial	30	1-Jun-19	30-Aug-19	28-Dec-19	27-Mar-20	448.5	180.3
GroupIIITrialX	Group III - Last Drug Trial	30	1-Aug-19	30-Oct-19	28-Mar-20	26-Jun-20	323.6	320.8
GroupIVTrialA	Group IV - First Drug Trial	30	1-Sep-19	30-Nov-19	29-Mar-20	27-Jun-20	261.1	322.6
GroupIVTrialX	Group IV - Last Drug Trial	30	1-Nov-19	30-Jan-20	30-Mar-20	28-Jun-20	135.0	332.0
	Total						2,767.3	535.6

These summaries should be enough to do any budgeting or other planning.

Given these reports as a basis, anyone familiar with Excel should be able to easily generate other reports.

9. Managing a Trial

Assuming that we have the above plan together, the next step is to consider what needs to be done as the studies start and continue to conclusions.

The spreadsheets for the plan should be saved and probably protected against being modified by unauthorized individuals. Then, another copy of the plan should be made and named with the current month as part of the filename, such as "Plan-March17.xls".

Actuals

The first step will be to collect the actual resources, dates, and costs that have been developed in the above plan. The "actuals" will probably come from several different sources;

Dates

The sites are typically responsible for the start and end of study execution. The sponsor will be responsible for the study start and end or completion of the clinical summary. Perhaps the best (and maybe the only) way to track the dates is through frequent meetings or other communications between the Sponsor and the sites.

Costs

Tracking monthly costs will probably require interaction with the financial departments of the sponsor and the site.

Resources

Tracking actual resources will involve "time-reporting" for those involved in the study. This can cause some issues. Some staff might object to having to report their time. Most of the people working on clinical trials will be "salaried" instead of "hourly". In your organization the terms might be "professional" vs "technical". Whatever the names it will be important to obtain estimates of the actual time spent working on a trial. This usually does not mean filling out daily time-sheets. In some cases each person can fill out a time-sheet once each month to "estimate" the time spent on each study. In some cases there might be an administrative assistant who could look over schedules and do the estimating.

A time sheet such as the following would suffice.

Project Management of Clinical Trials

Study Title	
Time Sheet for Month, Year	
Name	
Resource	

Department - Personnel
Nurse Resource	
Study Coordinator	
Investigator	
Lab Effort	
Pharmacy	
IT	
Accounting	
Other	

Other Monthly Costs
Drug Supplies	
Lab Processing	

Annual Fixed Costs
Other Computer	
Other Computer	
Other Personnel	
Other Procedures	

Obviously, a time sheet for each resource that lists the potential studies would also work.

If you retrieve this information for each resource and each study, then it will be possible to produce reports that show these "actuals" compared to the Plan.

Project Management of Clinical Trials

For example;

Nurse Resource Study Title	YTD Resource vs Actual ($k) Planned	Actual	Variance	Monthly Resource vs Actual ($k) Planned	Actual	Variance
First Drug Trial	5.0	3.0	2.0	1.0	1.0	0.0
Second Drug Trial	4.0	3.0	1.0	1.0	1.0	0.0
Third Drug Trial	3.0	3.0	0.0	1.0	1.0	0.0
Fourth Drug Trial	5.0	3.0	2.0	1.0	1.0	0.0
Fifth Drug Trial	2.0	3.0	(1.0)	1.0	1.0	0.0
Sixth Drug Trial	0.0	3.0	(3.0)	0.0	1.0	(1.0)
Seventh Drug Trial	0.0	3.0	(3.0)	0.0	1.0	(1.0)
Eighth Drug Trial	0.0	3.0	(3.0)	0.0	1.0	(1.0)
Total	19.0	24.0	(5.0)	5.0	8.0	(3.0)
	5.0					

Nurse Resource Study Title	YTD Costs vs Actual ($k) Planned	Actual	Variance	Monthly Cost vs Actual ($k) Planned	Actual	Variance
First Drug Trial	25.0	15.0	10.0	5.0	5.0	0.0
Second Drug Trial	20.0	15.0	5.0	5.0	5.0	0.0
Third Drug Trial	15.2	15.0	0.2	5.0	5.0	0.0
Fourth Drug Trial	25.0	15.0	10.0	5.0	5.0	0.0
Fifth Drug Trial	10.0	15.0	(5.0)	5.0	5.0	0.0
Sixth Drug Trial	0.0	15.0	(15.0)	0.0	5.0	(5.0)
Seventh Drug Trial	0.0	15.0	(15.0)	0.0	5.0	(5.0)
Eighth Drug Trial	0.0	15.0	(15.0)	0.0	5.0	(5.0)
Total	95.2	120.0	(24.8)	25.0	40.0	(15.0)

This report would hypothetically show the Nursing Resource for a given month. It shows the total estimated for each study in the plan and then the planned against actual for the month.

Given this information, it would then be possible to look into any studies where there is a large variance. In the case above, it looks like many of the studies were perhaps started early.

9.1 Study Start-up

The following activities need to be accomplished and completed before the study starts. That is, before patients can be seen.

Role	Sponsor	Site
Study Protocol	X	
CRF or eCRF	X	
ePRO	X	
IRB Approval	X	X
Patient Enrollment		X
Randomization	X	
Study Medications	X	X
Lab Setup		X
Special Equipment		?
Informed Consent		?

The study start can be delayed by any of the following;

- Failure to get signatures on some of the key documents such as Protocol, SAP, or IRB approval.
- Lack of adequate, properly labeled drug supply
- Lack of printed and distributed paper CRFs
- Lack of availability of Clinical Data Entry system
- One of the laboratories is not ready to process the samples.
- Lack of Patients available for the study.

9.2 Study Execution

Role	Sponsor	Site
Patient Enrollment		X
Study Visits		X
Randomization		X
Study Medication		X
Lab Results		X
Computer Resources	X	X
Special Equipment	X	X
Data Entry	X	X
Records Mgmt	X	X

Study Execution completion dates will typically be influenced by;

> The rate of patient enrollment – in some cases it may occur faster than expected and the study will finish early.
> Delays in patient attendance. If the patients simply do not live up to the schedule.
> Serious adverse events that cause the Safety Monitoring Board to terminate the study early.
> Positive results can also cause a study to be terminated early.

9.3 Study Close-out

Role	Sponsor	Site
Database Lock	X	X
Statistical Analyses	X	
Clinical Summary(s)	X	
Archive Records	X	X
Medication Accountability	X	X

Locking the database usually involves having the sponsor review the data in the database and then sending any outstanding issues such as erroneous or missing data to site for resolution. Most companies today are trying to have the sites enter the data directly when they are seeing the patient and the computer will raise any issues as the data are entered. This means the problems or issues are raised as the study is progressing and there are no issues to resolve when the last visit occurs.

The Statistical Analysis and the Clinical Summary are typically the sole responsibility of the sponsor.

Original records for the study often involve both the sponsor and the site. There will be records in both places and in some cases the same record may need to be accessible to both parties.

In most studies the medication has to be accounted for. Many of the medications are controlled substances and need to be controlled but it also may be necessary to verify the proper use of the medication during the trial.

Delays or other problems in this step can come from any of the Roles above, Delays in preparation of the Clinical Summary can be caused by any of the following.

Delays in locking the database
Unexpected Statistical results
Unexpected Clinical Results

The archiving of the records can seem straight-forward. The one thing that is often over-looked is that the records and the procedures need to be periodically tested. It is a good idea to test the retrieval when the records are archived and then again soon after the archival is in place. If it is tested fairly quickly, it might be possible to recover the records because not too much time has passed.

9.4 Making Adjustments to the Plan

Adjusting the plan is something that should be done monthly. Do make these adjustments the following is recommended;

1. Make a copy of the previous month's plan.

   Copy the previous month's plan to a new file with the month in the filename. For example, "Drugname-Feb 01". This will give you the option to compare different months if that becomes necessary.

2. Enter Actuals for the Month

   Enter the "Actuals" for that month and setup the necessary meetings and correspondence to review the Plan.

3. Review the Actuals vs Planned

   Go through any "large" deviations from the plan and decide on resolutions. It may be decided to not make a change this month, but monitor what goes on during the next month and then make a decision.

4. Make any Necessary Adjustments to the Plan

   Make any changes to the plan that might be necessary.

5. Publish the new Plan

   Distribute copies of the new plan to those required see it. Decide if more meetings or other monitoring might be necessary for the next month.

9.5 Making Changes to the Spreadsheets

Throughout the spreadsheets formulas have been used to

   Carry values on the "Defaults" spreadsheet forward
   Carry values on the "Standard" studies spreadsheets forward
   Use "$" where possible to hold values when entries are copied

It is recommended that changes to the spreadsheets should be done by someone with Excel experience.

9.6 Adding a new "Standard" Trial

A new standard trial can be added by simply copying one of the exiting trials and then making any required changes.

9.7 Deleting a Standard Trial

Any of the Standard Trials can be deleted by simply deleting the spreadsheet if there are no trials defined by copying that spreadsheet to a new Trial.

9.8 Adding a new Resource

All of the spreadsheets refer to the "Defaults" spreadsheet. If there is a resource that is not being used, simply change a resource that is not in use in the Defaults spreadsheet to the resource you need.

To add a new resource, start with the Defaults worksheet

> Insert a blank line below the last resource
> Copy the last resource
> Paste that Resource using the "keep formulas" option
> Make any necessary changes to the new resource

Go through each spreadsheet and

> Insert a blank line below the last resource
> Paste the new resource from the Defaults worksheet into the blank line

9.9 Adding a New Study

Copy one of the Standard worksheets to the new Study. Update the spreadsheet with the new study information.

If the studies are being grouped in the Summaries then the location of the study in with the other studies is important. If, for example, the new study is a Phase II study, then the worksheet needs to be stored in with the other Phase II studies.

Go through each of the Summary spreadsheets that list individual studies and add the new study by doing the following;

> Insert a blank line where you want the study
> Copy the entire line above it into that blank line using "Keep Formulas"
> Make any necessary changes to the Study name
> Change the corresponding entry in column A

Notes

10. Valid Processes

So you are probably asking yourself "What is a Valid Process as opposed to just a Process?" In this industry you will find that the "processes" as we are using them are supported by some "Procedure", so the two terms might be used interchangeably.

Process Validation is defined as the collection and evaluation of data, from the ***process design stage throughout production,*** which establishes scientific evidence that a process is capable of consistently delivering quality products.

There is a term that has become very unpleasant within computer circles in the Pharmaceutical industry. That term is "Validation" or the "V" – word. Many people argue that it really just increases cost and causes delays. In fact, if it is done correctly it does the opposite.

Now, some of this is "pay me now or pay me later". When working with computer systems we have known for about 55 years that these "validation" things are necessary for the success, and continued success of any computer system. Most other industries, aerospace, defense, and now the finance industry have learned to validate their systems. For some reason, the Healthcare Industry still is arguing "No, we don't have to do that".

10.1 Process Validation

There has been a lot of documentation and work with Process Validation.

In a 1978 guidance document the FDA defined process validation as follows;

Process Validation

> Establishing documented evidence that provides a high degree of assurance that a specific process will consistently produce a product meeting its predetermined specifications and quality attributes.

In a more recent guidance document (2011) the definition is;

> *Process Validation* is defined as the collection and evaluation of data, from the process design stage through commercial production, which establishes scientific evidence that a process is capable of consistently delivering quality product. Process validation involves a series of activities taking place over the lifecycle of the product and process.

This definition is particularly important because it introduces the notion of a Lifecycle. In Project Management a life cycle is a very important concept. It is particularly important when dealing with a computer system. The development and use of a computer system typically follows a Systems Development Lifecycle (SDLC) or more recently, a Systems Lifecycle (SLC).

If we look at the definition of Process Validation that appeared in the earlier (1987) document, there are several phrases in this definition that are important to understand by themselves.

Establishing Documented Evidence

There has to be "Documented Evidence". In other words, there has to be *documentation*. If there are any processes in your work that someone is saying "This does not need to be documented." **Be careful**. It is likely that it is against the law to use that process.

You will find that the one key to Compliance is "How are things Documented?" This documentation is a product of the process.

High Degree of Assurance

As you do your job you have to be able to measure how well you are doing. This was a key component to what W. E. Deming did in Japan. You have a responsibility to know if you are getting better or staying the same. No one, including the FDA requires that you do things perfectly all the time, but they do expect you to know how good you are.

Specific Process

A *systematic* series of actions directed to some end:

Everything we do should follow some "Process" the steps and important aspects of that process should be known, and can be documented.

Produce a Product

One of the key notions in all of this work is the production of something tangible (or electronic). If you go through a series of steps and do not produce anything you can "touch" be CAREFUL. This means you cannot prove that you did something the right way.

Meeting Predetermined

Specifications
Quality Attributes

> These specifications and quality attributes are known (and documented) before the process is performed. They will be updated and changed as the product/process is used.

10.2 Process Management and Project Management

How we do things?

Start with a simple lifecycle like the following;

Step 1 – Decide *What* to do.

Step 2 – Decide *How* to do it.

> *Note; It is not unusual to get these two reversed. Be careful, that can cause problems.*

Step 3 – Do what you decided, the way you decided. This should have some rules.

Step 4 – Evaluate what was done or produced to see if it is <u>What</u> you wanted and <u>How</u> you wanted it, according to the rules.

Step 5 – Use what you produced for what you wanted and manage changes.

Step 6 – When you are done with it, either store somewhere for later use or throw it away.

-- Notes --

Never buy a car you can't push.

11. Development of SOPs

As you might expect there are some general rules for the development of SOPs that make it possible to manage these documents. Obviously there can be exceptions to some of these but keep in mind what the text is recommending.

11.1 Identifying the SOP

When an SOP is displayed, either on paper or on a screen, each page or screen should have a header or footer something like the following to identify the specific SOP. This is important to the person executing the SOP but it is also important if the operator decides to print the page or the screen. This information will identify the specific SOP and step in the SOP.

Company Seal	Title:	ID: SOP-MMM-nn
Effective Date ___/___/___	Approved by: Title:	Page 1 of 3

Title: Have the complete, unique title for the SOP

ID: It is important to have a unique identifier for the SOP so that if it is referenced elsewhere there will be no question about identifying the correct SOP. Typically the ID is made up of two parts. The first is the unique identifier for the SOP, the second part is the "Version" number of the SOP. This number is incremented each time the SOP is changed. The products of the SOP will have a date associated with them. It is vital to know the date of the Product compared to the date of the SOP that produced it.

Approved by: This should identify the person and their title that is responsible for the SOP.

Page numbering: The page or screen number needs to be displayed with the total number of pages or screens in the SOP.

11.2 *History of Revisions*

It is important to identify the changes that have been made to the SOP over time. Any auditors and FDA inspectors believe that problems tend to occur when changes are being made. A table such as the following will typically appear on the first page or the last page of the SOP.

Version	Date	Change	Approved
001-AA	mm/dd/yyyy	Original Version	Initials or sign.

11.3 SOP Sections

There can be any number of different sections in an SOP depending on what the procedure is but the following should be in almost every SOP

Scope and Purpose

These sections should describe what areas and practices the SOP applies to. This is vital because you do not want someone; this includes an auditor or inspector, to apply the SOP in an area where it is not intended.

References

As you prepare the steps in the procedure there will be cases where the steps are already documented in a user manual or other document (inputs). The question will come up as to whether you should "copy" and "paste" from the other document into the SOP.

It is usually better to simply reference the other document, including its version number or date. If the other document changes it might get complicated trying to reproduce the instructions in the SOP.

Therefore, it is usually a good idea to specifically list any related documents. This includes other SOPS that are referenced in the SOP.

Glossary of Terms

Include a list of terms or abbreviations used in the SOP. Again, this is to avoid any possible confusion. This might also be a place where you want to reference a list of abbreviations in another document. The issue will be, what is the best way to keep the list updated accurately?

Procedure

Of course, there needs to be a Procedure section that lists the steps that are executed during the procedure.

Procedures can tend to be one of two types or one of two extremes. The first case might be a series of steps is executed to produce a single product that is then used.

The other extreme is where a series of steps is executed where each step is similar. For example, if a client walks in the door to a store, there might be series of steps each client goes through to obtain their desired product, or when a patent walks into a clinic or hospital they will be subjected to a series of tests. The series of tests and the order will depend on the particular symptoms and the results of earlier tests.

It is also often better to keep the steps short. Avoid writing long paragraphs to describe each step. One or two sentences for each step is probably best. If there needs to be a long explanation of what is to be done, it might be better to refer to another document and add a training step if necessary.

Products

The procedure needs to produce certain "Products". These are the Quality records.

They might be other documents, for example, specification for developing and supporting a computer system. The "product" produced might be a cure. The steps to obtain the product can be very different and produce a list of products – different test results.

In any case, as was mentioned earlier, be careful if the procedure produces no products.

Deviations

It is not unusual to find as you are executing the SOP that you need to deviate from it. There is some room for judgment when you find you need to deviate.

If it is necessary to change a few of the steps for some unanticipated reason, that could be classified as a deviation. If you get into it and the entire SOP needs to be changed, that is probably more than a "Deviation" and should require more attention.

When you get into an SOP and find that a couple steps need to be changed, it is not a problem if the "deviation" is documented and approved.

For example, If the 4th step says to collect a urine specimen but you cannot for some reason, you should have a field somewhere, perhaps a comment field, where you can document that you could not complete step 4, explain why, and have the action approved by someone.

What to do when a deviation occurs can either be documented in the SOP itself or in the SOP on SOPs.

11.4 Length and Detail

In general, an SOP should be relatively short. That is, no longer than 2 – 8 pages. If it gets longer than that it has been found that people won't really study them.

It is also a good idea to be careful about how much detail is included. Obviously you want to have enough detail so the person can follow the procedure but the detail can be referred to instead of included in the SOP.

Often the detail will change and you need to be sure the reference is to the accurate version but it can be a hassle to get SOPs approved so you don't want to be in a situation where the SOPs need to be approved every other day.

To help this some things to consider are;

> Don't use people's names, use Job Titles.
> Don't reference specific file names.

11.5 Contents

As was said earlier, reference other documentation that describes the detail. In general it is not good practice to cut-and-paste large sections of other documentation into the SOPs. The contents of the SOPs needs to be kept up-to-date. If you start cutting pasting sections of other documents, over time, the maintenance can become problematic.

11.6 Reviews

Review the SOPs on a regular basis, perhaps once a year or after any organizational, content, or procedural changes that might impact the execution of the procedure.

11.7 SOP on SOPs

Have one SOP that describes the material listed above and how to produce them.

12. Sample SOPs

Two templates follow below

> Standard Operating Procedure Template
> Information Systems Training Record

Standard Operating Procedure

SOP-001	Title: SOP Template	Version; 00A
Effective Date	Approved by;	
Applies to;		Page 1 of 2

Approvals

Name/Signature	Date

Annual Review Date:	By:

Version	Summary of changes

Standard Operating Procedure

SOP-001	Title: SOP Template	Version; 00A
Effective Date	Approved by;	
Applies to;		Page 2 of 2

1. Purpose

Describe the reason for the procedure and what products are produced.

2. Scope

Describe which areas and which practices are covered by this SOP and, if necessary, which areas are not covered.

3. Referenced Documents

Doc ID	Title	Date

4. Glossary/Definitions

Term	Definition

5. Procedure

Describe the process being documented in a step-by-step manner. Indicate where documentation that can be audited or inspected is produced.

6. Appendices

ttach or reference templates, or other documents that are used in the Procedure. Include the word "SAMPLE" in the water mark or footnote.

Standard Operating Procedure

SOP-001	Title: Information Systems Training Records	Version; 00A
Effective Date	Approved by;	
Applies to;		Page 1 of 3

Approvals

Name/Signature	Date

Annual Review Date:	By:

Version	Summary of changes

Standard Operating Procedure

SOP-001	Title: Information Systems Training Records	Version; 00A
Effective Date	Approved by;	
Applies to;		Page 2 of 3

INFORMATION SYSTEMS TRAINING RECORDS

PURPOSE

This SOP describes the method of documenting the training of personnel in this department.

2.0 SCOPE

Any personnel involved in computer systems that are covered by validation guidelines must have adequate training. The training may include both computer usage and familiarity with the application system.

3.0 TRAINING RECORDS

A file will be maintained for each employee that documents the training and qualification of each employee. Each file will contain a CV of each employee's qualifications.

In addition, a list of all training received by each person in the department will be maintained in the same files (sample in Attachment A:). It will be the responsibility of each person to describe the training they have received and the dates it took place since the date of the CV.

This list should be updated as soon as possible after each course, but in any event, once each year (by January 31) the secretary will distribute to each employee his or her training list for them to update for the previous year. This is to be completed within 30 days and returned to the department manager for approval.

Both the employee and the manager will initial each training course on the list and return the list to the files.

If a certificate or other documentation exists for the course, a copy should be included in the file but is not required.

Standard Operating Procedure

SOP-001	Title: Information Systems Training Records	Version; 00A
Effective Date	Approved by;	
Applies to;		Page 3 of 3

Attachment A; Training Record

Name _____

Proc. No.	Title	Required?	If Yes, Understand and will follow	Signature/Date
	Change Control	☐ Yes ☐ No	☐ Yes ☐ No	
	Systems Development Life Cycle	☐ Yes ☐ No	☐ Yes ☐ No	
	Qualification of IT Systems	☐ Yes ☐ No	☐ Yes ☐ No	
	Qualification Master Plan	☐ Yes ☐ No	☐ Yes ☐ No	
		☐ Yes ☐ No	☐ Yes ☐ No	
		☐ Yes ☐ No	☐ Yes ☐ No	
		☐ Yes ☐ No	☐ Yes ☐ No	
		☐ Yes ☐ No	☐ Yes ☐ No	
		☐ Yes ☐ No	☐ Yes ☐ No	
		☐ Yes ☐ No	☐ Yes ☐ No	

-- **Notes** –

-- Notes --

Eat a live toad in the morning and nothing worse will happen to you the rest of the day.

13. If All Else Fails

I will say that from time to time I pray. I won't go into a lot of detail but there is a line in one of the prayers that goes

"Save us from the Fires of Hell"

Now that is probably not a bad plea regardless of your spiritual orientation, but I noticed at one point that I had replaced one of the words.

As you might guess from the previous chapters that virtually all of the documentation mentioned exists in files of some kind. They might be paper or electronic or some combination. It turned out that the line I had been actually saying, probably for many months was

"Save us from the Files of Hell"

Now after some thought I decided this was probably a much better prayer anyway.

I guess if you are having trouble doing compliance, don't be afraid to ask for help, wherever that help might be.

Appendix A - Quality Management.

The following diagram is from some earliier ISO 9000 documentation 1).

1. World Health Organization and Clinical and Laboratory Standards Institute, *SUPPLEMENT TO THE LABORATORY QUALITY MANAGEMENT SYSTEM TRAINING TOOLKIT, Module 16 - Documents and records.*

It helps to put some of this in perspective.

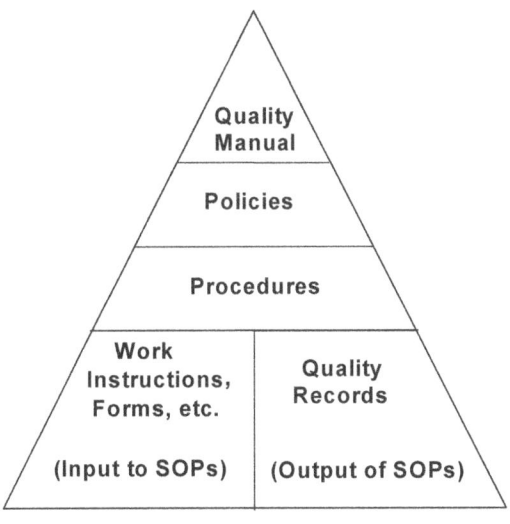

Quality Manual

> This is a document that describes the company's Quality Organization. It will discuss the role of Quality Assurance in the company as well as the responsibilities that each department has to quality.

Policies

> Generally, policies are 1 – 2 pages of high level, somewhat "apple pie and the flag", commitment to a concept. The concept might be to satisfy certain regulations or business practices.

Procedures

> The Procedures are a more detailed discussion explaining how to implement the policies and processes (SOP).

Below that there tends to be two types of documents:

> The documents that form the <u>input to the SOPs</u> will typically be the documentation such as; the Work Instructions, Manuals, Regulations, Operator's Guides, templates, or other more detailed documentation that will be referenced in the Procedures. These will lead to Processes to implement the policies. The documentation of these processes will typically be much larger. They might be "Work Instructions", computer system manuals, and other more lengthy descriptions of how to implement the policies
>
> The second set of documents is the <u>output from the SOPs</u> – the "deliverables". These are also referred

to as *Quality Records*. These are the documents that will be audited *against* the other documents. These are the "Evidence" for compliance.

There are four words that are used in what we all do. They all play a role in Compliance. It is vital that you and your organization have your own definitions for these words. It will also be important for you to understand how they map to similar words in the various regulations, guidance documents, and other documentation.

The four words are;

> Process
> Project
> Procedure
> Product

In all four cases we will be using the noun versions of these words.

If one goes to Internet and searches these four words you will find a large variety of definitions. In one case it actually says "there are 190 definitions of the word Project".

Based on that, the following four definitions have been chosen for use here.

> Process – A series of actions or steps taken in order to achieve a particular end.
> Project – A temporary endeavor undertaken to create a unique product or service
> Procedure – A particular course or mode of action.
> Product – A good, idea, method, information, object or service created as a result of a process and serves a need or satisfies a want.

Quality Assurance

The additional term for use is the following;

> Write down What you are supposed to do and How you do it.
> Follow those procedures
> Study what has happened to assure that you are doing What you are supposed to do and How you are supposed to do it (QC)
> If there is a problem, figure out how to fix it and "Improve the Process"
> Must be Pro-Active. You can't wait until something "breaks" (QA)

A Processes

At the top we have Processes. These will typically be a high-level description of what is to be done. They might also be called a "Policy".

We should be able to divide our workload into a set of "Processes" that we perform – the "Divide and Conquer Concept". Sometimes this can be a challenge.

Some of our processes might be simple cases where there are a handful of simple steps. In other cases our Process might have "Sub-Processes".

There will also be the case that some of the processes have dependencies between them where, for example, one has to finish before another one can start.

It is important to develop an understanding of the Processes and their relationships when you start to work on Project Management.

Some of the processes might come with lengthy descriptions of what to do. This can be very helpful but typically the readers will not read the whole document or there can be sections that are too general to be very helpful.

We are considering Clinical Research as a set of Processes that we use to produce various treatments for different illnesses.

As was mentioned earlier, you can define the processes as broadly as you like. For example, some processes might be

> Implement a computer system for tracking all serious adverse events.
> Implement a process for budgeting and tracking costs and resources for all projects in the company or division of a company.
> Conduct a Clinical Trial on Drug X
> Record all necessary medical information when seeing a patient – whatever manual or computer systems might be necessary. Include not only the observation but who made the observation, when, using what instrument, and so on.
> Record daily attendance, including times of arrival and departure.

Obviously there is room for judgment in some of these examples. The first example; implementing a computer system, could be one Process, but Conducting a Clinical Trial could be multiple processes if desired. The study setup – Defining the data entry, identifying the sites, could be one process. Study Execution – seeing patients could be another process.

Recording medical information could be one process for a clinic or hospital where the project might involve one Project for each area with the hospital.

Project Management of Clinical Trials

It could also be multiple processes, one for each area within the hospital where then each Process might be one Procedure.

Recording medical information could be one process for a clinic or hospital where the *process* might involve one **Procedure** for each area with the hospital.

Process – Record Patient Information
Procedure 1 – Cardiac Unit
Procedure 2 – Pediatric Unit
Procedure 3 – Geriatric Unit
- - - -
Procedure X – Special Unit

Time

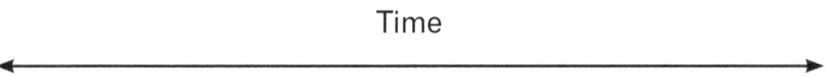

It could also be multiple processes, one for each area within the hospital where then each **Process** might be one **Procedure**.

Process – Cardiac Unit
Procedure 1 – Cardiac Unit
Process – Pediatric Unit
Procedure 2 –
Process – Geriatric Unit
Procedure 3 –
- - - -
Process – Special Unit
Procedure X –

Time

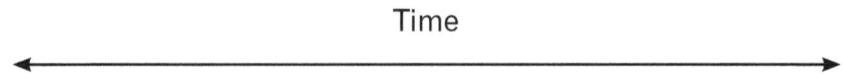

It is up to your organization to determine which definition works best.

When you are executing a process it is very important to understand the products produced. It might be an interesting exercise to ask those involved to describe the products being produced.

If there is not absolute agreement on what the products are then there is the potential for large problems.

Some Exceptions

As you can see above in some cases the project continues to exist after the Procedures are put in use. This is to provide continued support and Change Control – Which is also a relatively large issue with regulated processes.

In some cases the project part ends and any support, maintenance, or change control is covered with the Procedures.

How you decide to structure the work described here will depend on your company's Best Practices, the Applicable Regulations, your Products, and your Organization.

In order to focus on complying with regulations we are going to go through three concepts that constitute the heart of Compliance.

1. What is a Valid Process?

    If we are going to get in compliance, everything we do has to be viewed as a "Process", a series of steps that will yield some result(s) - products. The steps in these processes are the procedures that presumably reflect what our company wants us to be doing.

    The steps should be approved by your management.

2. What are Quality Assurance and Quality Control?

The American Society for Quality (ASQ) defines these as;

> **Assurance:** The act of giving confidence, the state of being certain or the act of making certain.
> **Quality Assurance:** The planned and systematic activities implemented in a quality system so that quality requirements for a product or service will be fulfilled.
> **Control:** An evaluation to indicate needed corrective responses; the act of guiding a process in which variability is attributable to a constant system of chance causes.
> **Quality Control:** The observation techniques and activities used to fulfill requirements for quality.

Quality Assurance in our context is really just studying periodically to see (and to document) if, by following our procedures, we are producing the desired products in the desired way. If not, there are ways to make necessary corrections and continue (CAPA).

B Personnel

One of the most important aspects of project management, especially in this environment is the personnel and their responsibilities. Many of the regulations assign specific responsibilities to those doing the work. The training these personnel have received is also very important. It is not unusual to have an auditor or inspector asked to see someone's training records.

C Projects

We will be viewing each clinical trial as a "Project". Given that, there will be some related activities that can also be viewed as a project, or perhaps a "Sub-project". References like the Project Management Institute Body of Knowledge (PMBOK) and the IEEE Software Engineering Standards will be very helpful.

The Projects are endeavors undertaken to create a unique product, service, or procedure.

Some of the Projects will be temporary and produce a single result and then are closed. Other projects such as the development of a computer system will likely have a maintenance and support phase that will exist for the life of the system.

The projects will have "Procedures" that describe what is done and how to do it. These will be Standard Operating Procedures (SOPs). The SOPs will produce "Products" that are the things needed to do our work. The products will be Documentation, Logs of activities, Test scripts, and the other "Evidence" that the processes are being fulfilled accurately.

-- Notes --

The End

CPSIA information can be obtained
at www.ICGtesting.com
Printed in the USA
LVHW090837220820
663894LV00006B/73/J